The New ADD
in Adults Workbook

The New ADD in Adults Workbook

A Different Way of Thinking

Lynn Weiss, Ph.D.

TAYLOR TRADE PUBLISHING
Lanham • New York • Dallas • Boulder • Toronto • Oxford

Published by Taylor Trade Publishing
An imprint of The Rowman & Littlefield Publishing Group, Inc.
4501 Forbes Boulevard, Suite 200
Lanham, Maryland 20706

Distributed by National Book Network

ISBN 1-58979-248-3 (pbk. : alk. paper)

∞™ The paper used in this publication meets the minimum requirements of American
National Standard for Information Sciences—Permanence of Paper for Printed Library
Materials, ANSI/NISO Z39.48-1992.

Contents

Acknowledgments

The first acknowledgement I wish to make for this book is to the many folks in Dallas, Texas, in the early 1990s who spent time and energy to learn about their own ADD characteristics and what it would take to stay true to themselves while "making it" in the majority culture. We met together in small groups over a number of years, ferreting out many ways to survive and grow with an ADD style of brain construction. Without each of you, my work with this subject would have never progressed to the level it has.

Reality struck with the actual writing of this book. That's where the Rowman & Littlefield (Taylor) staff has helped me fashion the material into a readable unit. First thanks go to Janet Harris and Camille Cline, my editors, Rick Rinehart, editor in chief, and Stephen Driver, production editor who have stood by my side, guided me, and run interference when needed. Thanks, ladies—I truly appreciate you.

Thanks, too, to the many other Rowman & Littlefield folks who made sure that the book was finished with a quality look and opened the doors so it can find its way in the hands of those who can make use of it.

On a personal level, there are my dear friends Judy and Mike Weinrobe, who graciously turned their spare bedroom over to me for my editorial trips to Dallas. My Bastrop friends and colleagues, Tiffany Green and Fleeta Cunningham, writing cohorts who listened to my tales of woe, soothed my tense brow, and rejoiced in the completion of this manuscript. The Bastrop Writers' Group cheered me on and let me test the material further. And finally, my son, Aaron, who is always willing to take a minute to answer a computer question or burn a CD. Thanks one and all

Introduction

In this book I talk about a brain diversity issue that is simply a stylistic set of traits passed from generation to generation through a family line. Attention Deficit Disorder (ADD), a term I'll use in this book synonymously with Attention Deficit Hyperactivity Disorder (ADHD), is a perfectly normal style of brain construction. It is not a pathological condition to be diagnosed and treated. I am not talking about Acquired ADD such as results from diet, head injuries, cocaine or alcohol abuse, metal poisoning, birth defects, or allergies.

I've seen many of us lose touch with the usefulness of our innate ADD style because our natural style didn't fit the expectation of the world around us. We have resources that go unrecognized—resources that we can use to achieve our goals. Instead of feeling hopeless to get our work, studies, and relationships *right*, we can learn to act in ways to reach our goals *effectively*.

We all have to learn to go about the job of discovering our inner resources. Then we must find ways to use them on our own behalf. Sometimes we have to find ways to heal the feelings of hopelessness and helplessness that we learned as a result of not being tuned into our hidden resources. These lessons make up the themes woven through this book.

Many of us no longer see our innate talents. We don't recognize and have not received appropriate training to use our natural skills and talents. We have underachieved and been hurt as a result, and we've often given up trying "to get things right."

The skills in this book were originally forged with people who have a high number of ADD attributes. I've come to realize, however, that many of the issues that emerged for them are issues many more people experience to some degree. Each of us must find out how our own brain is made. We must be sure we find the right places to utilize our resources so we may use them positively. We must, above all, refine our thinking tools to accomplish outcomes that make sense for each of us and maximize our effectiveness.

Then, strong in our own right, we can team up with others who have a different constellation of skills. Together we become unbeatable.

THE BASIC FRAMEWORK FOR THIS BOOK

You will find three themes woven throughout this book. Many of the suggestions are geared to help you recognize and support the innate brainstyle attributes with which you are born—the ones that reflect your greatest strengths.

But when your innate strengths are pressed into learning and living environments that don't fit them, you end up hurt. As a result, you will need to find ways to heal those hurts so you can use your natural skills effectively.

Finally, you will discover ways to accommodate your natural skills and interests to situations that don't fit you. The trick here is to do what you need to do without damaging yourself in the process.

THEME ONE: HIDDEN RESOURCES OF THE TRUE YOU

You have a natural style of brain construction—one with which you were born. I call that style the True You. It is from the core of your True Self that the hidden resources, previously dormant or disallowed, will be encouraged to come into full bloom. In this book, you will be encouraged and helped to recognize and respect your hidden resources. What lay previously undetected or underdeveloped can be embraced and used in your personal and work life for the benefit of all.

The True You is the unwarped, unjudged, unwounded, natural you. All of the original innate skills, talents, attributes, and gifts with which you were born are available to you to use as you choose. In this book, I'll ask you to focus on the way in which you think, act, and express yourself. I'll talk about what you like and how you can go about reaching the goals that are important to you in a way that fits your natural bent. I'll look at how to make use of your brain in ways that can provide you with both happiness and success.

You'll learn to recognize what fits you by noticing feelings of enthusiasm and hesitation within yourself. You will be drawn to activities and situations that are right for you, that support your natural skills, and that provide you with a sense that you can reach your potential. In contrast, you will begin to learn to recognize your hesitation to engage in activities and situations that don't naturally fit you and that are not good for you. As you honor this wisdom within yourself, your life path will smooth out. Your journey will belong to you. Your pleasure will increase. And you will come to know meaningful success.

THEME TWO: THE WOUNDED YOU

No matter how you were raised or what your style of brain construction, you undoubtedly bumped into situations that did not fit your natural style of learning and working. You are likely to feel bruised as a result. You also probably learned to disregard your natural resources for learning and accomplishing things so that they went underground, out of your conscious awareness.

The result means you have been hurt, though often unintentionally. Now you'll learn how you can heal those hurts. Then you'll be able to effectively reconnect with your True Self. You'll become aware of the right environment for you—one that serves the needs of your True Self so you can retrieve your lost skills and talents

How Wounding Happens

In today's world, there are three typical contexts from which you are likely to have suffered the wounding.

Socialization

All societies have beliefs about what are right and proper ways for its members to behave. When these beliefs do not reflect the reality and diversity of how humans are made, wounding results. If, for example, sitting still in school is thought to indicate a high level of socialization, then those of us who learn by being active will be hurt. It's that simple.

The Learning of Harmful Beliefs

Wounding happens when a person believes there is only one acceptable way to be, to do, to think, or to live. All other ways, the result of different innate skills and talents, are considered flawed. Previously, beliefs have been the business of religion, but the damage done by beliefs has now spread throughout medicine, education, employment, and the legal system. ADD/ADHD (Attention Deficit Disorder/Attention Deficit Hyperactive Disorder), "the disability," and its placement in the Americans with Disabilities category is an example of such a belief.

The Leveling of Judgments

If a person with the untapped resources of his True Self is judged to be pathological because his natural way of doing things doesn't fit the current social model, the person is wounded by virtue of being judged. This applies to people labeled with Attention Deficit Disorder. They are even said to have a medical problem, are often denied an education that fits their brain construction, and are judged for work by standards that preclude their showing what they can do.

In addition to being thwarted from using their natural talents, they must be labeled *disabled* in order to be given an opportunity to achieve. Further damage comes from having to raise their hands and say, "There is something *wrong* with me."

Secondary Wounding

Additional damage occurs when a person buys into the belief that says his or her innate way is wrong. Self-depreciation results and continues damaging a person as long as the belief persists.

If you are required to do something that doesn't fit you and you resist, complain, react, or become depressed, anxious, clumsy, or indecisive, you are likely to be scolded, chastised, or furthered labeled because you've reacted. When you resist, you may be called oppositional. When you complain, you may be called argumentative. When you cry or become depressed, you are called symptomatic. When you become anxious, you are given a pathological label and medication to deal with your symptoms.

But these secondary symptoms are only the result of being pressured or forced to do something that doesn't fit you in the first place—something that is out of alignment with what is in the best interest of your True Self. Then when you are additionally labeled with behavioral or emotional problems, you are wounded a second time.

This latter wounding of people with diverse brainstyles does not need to happen. The secondary problems or symptoms are not inherently a part of the original True Self and its innate brainstyle. The behaviors and feelings are only indicators that something is amiss with the relationship between an individual's way and the environments in which that person is living. Instead of the person needing to change, the environment may need to be changed. One's True Self needs to be saved from being required to do what doesn't fit. Then the secondary symptoms disappear.

THEME THREE: THE ACCOMMODATING YOU

Even when you have mastered your True Self and know the kinds of settings in which you can optimally function, you will encounter the imperfect world of everyday life. Living in an imperfect world means you will not always be able to find a fit between your natural ways and the environments you face. But you can learn skills to bridge the differences between your innate skills and the expectations placed on you. And you can do this without hurting yourself further.

Accommodating to Your Environment

As you become aware of your True Self, you will learn to recognize how well your surroundings fit you. You'll become attuned to beliefs that honor you. At the same time, you will continue to respond the best you can until you can do something to make those changes.

On a personal level, you will be able to make plans, aligning your life with the needs of your True Self. But such moves take time. Take, for example, a move to self-employment. This will require time to adjust your finances, family obligations, and inner courage before you can actually make the step. You may also need to acquire some new skills. While you are acquiring the tools you need to make such moves, you will learn to accommodate to your current situation so you are not further wounded.

In this book, you will find both the light at the end of the tunnel and illumination as you travel to that light. Know that you are perfect the way you are naturally constructed. Know that your untapped resources are desperately needed not only by you but also by the society in which you live. But also know that there is usually a considerable lag between any new way to look at a situation and the actual changing of society to accommodate that new perspective.

THE REWARDS OF DIVERSITY

As you get to know yourself, your strengths and weaknesses, and what to do about them, you can become aware of what you need in order to allow those strengths to flourish. You become aware of what expectations and situations fit you and which don't. And you then are able to make choices that are in your best interest. Once you're in tune with your True Self, yoiu'll begin to see a style of pursuit that fits you best as you strive toward a goal. Even when expectations upon you and requirements of a goal do not fit you, you'll be able to find ways to succeed that do not set you up for failure. You can rationally measure the differences between your natural self and the requirements of the situation and escape self-depreciation. You then learn to accommodate to situations that don't much fit you without being maimed in the process.

With perspective, you will no longer hold yourself to impossible expectations. Instead, you'll find pathways to achieve the outcomes you desire in ways that use your strengths. No longer do you need to be hounded by shame, guilt, and feelings of inadequacy. The prize will be the good feelings you have about yourself and successful utilization of the best of what you innately have to offer any situation.

NATURAL RESOURCES

Let's look at the skills that often go untapped in today's world. People with lots of creative, right-brained, natural ability will recognize and feel at ease with these resources. This can be called the ADD-way. Others with a more linear way of doing things may not wish to utilize these ADD-style skills, but may find knowledge of them helpful in recognizing how others see the world and approach tasks.

Either way, knowing what these resources are gives all of us a balanced palette of skills when we encounter brainstyle differences on our way to accomplishing goals.

Skill 1: We Have the Ability to See the Big Picture

Many of us see the big picture before we see or make use of any of the details that make it up. Usually creative by nature, big-picture people often see a complete vision of what we want to achieve before we start moving toward our goals. In fact, we don't travel well to any goal unless we are provided with the overall big picture to begin with.

Skill 2: We Think in Terms of How Things Function

If we are to know how to proceed toward a goal, we must know its purpose. How is this goal to be used? Rather than seeing the details that make up the task, we see the function the details play. Then we can know the steps to take to achieve the goal.

Skill 3: We Pay Attention to the Patterns and Relationships within the Big Picture

Our focus of attention tends to be on the relationships between details rather than on the details themselves. We first see the interconnections and patterns that are formed between things rather than the elements that make them up.

Skill 4: We Express High Levels of Activity— Physical, Mental, Emotional, and Verbal

Naturally invested with lots of energy, we learn, create, and produce best when we are active. Our innate skills seek environments for expression that allow us to be physically active and verbally expressive. Our minds are curious and exploring and often work at lightning speed. After all, we see the big picture first so we don't need to slowly progress from one detail to another in order to reach that completed picture. We skate throughout the big picture on the patterns and interconnections between the details, moving quickly to a sense of the total function of everything that leads to our goals. We're also aided by our rapid awareness of the patterns that give us early clues about the journey we are taking.

Skill 5: We Learn by Doing (Kinesthetic Learning)

We naturally learn through the process of doing something rather than by reading or listening *about* whatever we are learning. We write a book to learn to write. We don't learn to write a book by studying about writing a book, doing exercises, worksheets, or taking exams so we can then write a book. We are totally and completely able to learn any subject or body of professional material, no matter how complex, by utilizing kinesthetic learning. That's why the apprenticeship model works well for us.

Skill 6: We Have an Inner Locus of Perception and Control

Our worldview comes from within ourselves. Our ability to organize, work with time and timing, maintain control over our behavior, and do whatever we need to do is idiosyncratically guided from within ourselves rather than from outside. We know and sense and can learn to live in a responsible way that yields the same results achieved by our more linear counterparts if we follow what *feels right* to us. We know what to do by listening to our inner drumbeat, not by using a template produced outside of ourselves into which we are expected to fit.

Skill 7: We Have a High Level of Sensitivity

Our sensitivity is felt through our senses: sight, sound, taste, smell, and touch as well as intuition. Extremely empathetic, our sensors are finely calibrated. Liken us to the dog that hears sounds not perceived by the human ear. We sense at a level that not all people have available to them. We are empathic and responsive to our environments. We also can be wounded when others do not see or sense the source of the wounding, yet we experience it nonetheless. When a companion has a feeling such as anger, we know it even if the person is unaware of it or denies it. Many of us are psychic though we may not be comfortable with this skill or may not purposely use it.

Skill 8: We Are Responsive

Because we are so sensitive and tend to act kinesthetically when attempting to reach a goal, we tend to be seen as reactive. With a wide range of emotions, readily experiencing joy and pain, we often express our feelings and do something about situations that others do not even know exist.

Skill 9: We Have a Strong Sensing Capability

We tend to think first through our ability to sense what is going on rather than by thinking about something. We simply *know*, having an inner sensory vision, experience, or intuition. We often feel the sensing physically in our bodies. Once we've perceived an event on a sensory level, we can decide what to do in response. We even store information using this mechanism rather than by categorizing according to the labels in more general use.

Skill 10: We Resonate to the Rhythmic Timing of Nature

Rather than responding to an arbitrary scheme to keep track of time, we tend to use natural rhythms and our own internal timing to get things done. We can apply this skill to a project or to getting the rest our bodies need. We may work at night and sleep in the daytime. We may naturally eat at times that vary from a three-meal-a-day schedule. We rarely break projects down into equal time segments in order to get them done by a certain time, but rather work when we *feel* creative and don't work when we feel unwilling or hesitant. When our innate timing is allowed to blossom and we are trained to recognize it, we always get things done *on time*.

These are at least some of the skills of the ADD-way—a storehouse of attributes that can contribute handsomely to the achievement of any goal.

BRAINSTYLE DIVERSITY

There is not one right way to be. There is a wide range of variation in the way in which humans are constructed. We all have our unique perspectives of life, shaped by our innate physical construction. Our bodies and brains look and function differently. Our experiences vary widely, so how in the world can we be expected to do things in the same way?

The skills of the ADD-way are different from the skills of the linear brainstyle. Neither is superior or inferior to the other. But they are completely different and each is little understood by those not constructed with the mental hardware to see or use them. In a judgment-free environment, however, representatives from the diverse sides of the brainstyle continuum can work in tandem, enhancing each other's assets.

Each of us is born with certain strengths and limitations. One person is expansively creative while another makes detailed records of transactions. A third has characteristics of both and is able to bring her creative expressions into orderly presentation for all people to enjoy. No one style of being made is better than another. Every strength has an up side and a down side. It is for each of us to realize what these strengths are in ourselves and to use them to advantage.

The honoring of diversity—whether it is in relation to skin color, sexual identity, age, or brain construction—is a must if we are to become healthy human beings and our society is to become one in which variation yields wholeness. In this context, each of us plays a valuable role no matter how we are made. But before we can honor the diversity brought by variations in brainstyle, we must recognize both its existence and its value for the society as a whole. We must learn when to rely on our own skills and when to team with others to produce a broader outcome.

This book is dedicated to assisting each of us to be all we can be and to contribute the best we have to offer for the good of our society as we learn a different way of thinking.

How to Use This Book

The New ADD in Adults Workbook is designed to have two authors: me *and* you, the user. It is, after all, a *work*book, which means each reader will answer its questions in a personal way. I'll lay out the principles I've observed that make up the ADD-way—principles that reflect the themes of that way.

The new workbook is designed to be used in one of two ways. It can be used as a companion "how to" book to the fourth edition of *ADD in Adults* or as a stand-alone book that will provide you with a different way to experience ADD. Either use will allow you to make the adjustments you need to make to live successfully, as you are.

Both books take into account the three themes of the True You, the Wounded You, and the Accommodating You. The workbook guides you to find, honor, and expand the attributes of your True Self, attributes that will lead to the kind of life you desire to live. Some of the sections in the workbook will help you to heal wounded parts of yourself that have blocked your access to the expression of your True Self. It will also help you prevent further wounding at the hands of ignorance and unintentional abuse. And, finally, this workbook will show you ways to survive, without further wounding, the requirements of settings that don't naturally fit you as you journey to the goal of building a life that reflects the True You. The Accommodating You will learn how to navigate these rough waters and make your journey as pain-free as possible.

This book is divided into several sections so that you can easily find areas to work on that interest you. Trust yourself as you decide what to work on. You can work on the sections alone, with a partner, or in a group. Again, trust your sense of what to do.

Start wherever you want. You do not need to use the workbook in any special order. Feel free to be creative in your approach. On the other hand, you may wish to impose a structure on your workbook experience by starting at the beginning and moving through chapter by chapter. Skip items that are not a problem for you. Take time with items that cause you lots of trouble. In fact, go back over these items several times until you integrate the ideas and your behavior becomes automatic. Sometimes this never happens and that's okay, too. If you need prompting periodically, simply return to the workbook for a reminder.

No one knows as well as you do what is bothering you, causing you trouble, or requiring your attention. It's up to you whether you choose to work on a tough area or begin with something small and easier to deal with.

If at any time you feel anxious while using the materials, it is all right to set them aside. Your emotions may be attempting to tell you that you're trying to deal with something prematurely. Sometimes your anxiety indicates that there is more for you to face or work with than your vulnerability is ready to encompass. In that case, you may wish to consult with a counselor to help you get through it. Again, trust you judgment.

Above all, know that you'll come away from this workbook experience with new insights and skills. You will gain strength on all fronts for yourself and in relation to those with whom you work and live. You will be able to more effectively make use of your ADD style of brain construction so you can better reach your dreams and live your life the way you want.

❶

Organizing in New Ways

Everyone can organize, but we don't all do it in the same way. It doesn't matter whether we're talking about managing details, keeping track of volumes of numbers and letters, breaking projects into manageable steps that guarantee completion, or making efficient and responsible use of our time.

Yet the skills needed to accomplish these tasks elude many of us. As a result, we come to believe we are *dis*organized. And we are, when we try to organize in ways that don't fit us. As a result, questions arise such as "What's wrong with me?" and "Am I not trying hard enough?"

To understand what's happening, let's remember the purpose of organization: to be able to retrieve things and manage a flow of work that will get us to a goal of our choosing. How we do it and what our process of organization looks like is not the issue. Given this freedom, we may discover we have a perfectly workable system. If, however, organization is supposed to mean alphabetized labels, file cabinets with papers out of sight, clean surfaces, and goals arrived at one step at a time, we may fail abjectly and be branded incompetent.

Our success at organization depends upon following organizational processes that fit our individualistic ways of using our innate brain construction. Sometimes training is needed to guide this process, but the training also must fit our style of thought. We must recognize that there are as many ways to organize as there are individual styles of brain construction. These alternative styles are what this section is about.

The True You will contain its own workable form of organization—ways that will easily allow you to achieve your goals. Many of the ones covered in this section have been developed by watching what works for creative, analog-processing, kinesthetic people.

You will also find continual encouragement to take what pleases you from these suggestions. What doesn't, I encourage you to lay aside, so you avoid further wounding from yet one more approach that doesn't fit you. On occasion, you'll be given suggestions for the Accommodating You so that you can make do until changes in your environment can be accomplished. The Accommodating You will find a path that prevents wounding while getting you where you want to go.

Remember, everyone has a natural pattern of organization within. Let's begin to find yours.

GETTING THE BEST OF CLUTTER

Question:

Do you Struggle with Clutter?

Why This Happens:

- When the True You is a creative, hands-on, big-picture person, you are likely to have many things that you are doing—lots of "somethings" to do.
- Out of sight is out of mind, so your "somethings" have to be visible if they are to get attended to.
- You may wish to creatively use something you've saved in the future. That's what creativity means—making variations on a theme so that every thing, event, or product is different from earlier models.
- When the "stuff" you're trying to organize is paper, you may need to read what is on the paper before knowing what to do with it—a very time-consuming activity.
- Reading, coming up with categories in which to file the paper, and step-by-step sorting of the paper is boring.
- Fear of not having resources at hand to meet an assignment or so that you can recall facts or details may lead you to keep everything, especially if you've been embarrassed, criticized, or teased in the past.

Problems You Face Because of Clutter:

- Clutter: deep piles of papers and "things" without a system for finding what you need in the clutter.
- Wasted time
- Frustration for yourself and others
- The appearance of irresponsibility

Your Goal:

To find a system that honors your style of brain construction so you can succeed at finding what you need when you need it and to have some personal and work areas that appear socially acceptable to others.

What Not To Do:

Do not get down on yourself for the way your space looks.

Your Work:

1. Analyze why your space is the way it is.
   I believe my space is cluttered because

   _____
   _____
   _____ .

2. What are you willing to do about it?

   _____
   _____

3. Check to see what emotional residue is left over from years of failure to "be organized." Make a list of your feelings and past experiences about organizing.
   My past experiences about organizing and how I felt about them are _____

   _____
   _____ .

4. Questions to ask yourself before you start to organize:

   Am I afraid I won't be able to accomplish the job?   _____yes
                                                         _____no
   Do I know how to proceed?   _____yes
                                                         _____no
   Am I able to find things just fine?   _____yes
                                                         _____no

   Are there any other reasons why I feel I can't or don't want to change the way I now organize? _____

   _____ .

5. Now you're ready to actually begin sorting and organizing. You will need to sort by the way in which something functions rather than by what it is called. For example, if you're cleaning off your desk, you might make categories for different things you find there.
   Supplies (pens, erasers)
   Writing stock (scratch paper, printer paper)
   Other supplies _____
   Place your supplies near where you are going to use them.
   Projects that need to be kept together could be divided into:

Active projects: Each active file needs to go in a separate pile that is kept out in the open so you can see it. Color-code each project so it has its own color. Place a piece of paper on the top using that color and use paper clips or stickers with that project's color. Label the file with the working name of the project.

References: Put them in the same stack as the active file next to whatever they are going to be used with. You might even clip them together using a sticker that's color-coded to match the associated project. Place a big "R" on the sticker, noting it's a reference.

Inactive projects: These are projects that have been completed or set aside for the time being. Make up category labels that associate them with either the function of the project or some easily recalled activity with which they were associated. If you use a name as a label, you are likely to fail to remember that name at a later time.

6. After you try the methods under #5, evaluate what you like about each and how you'd like to modify them.
   I like _____.
   I will try changing _____.
7. If you need a place to meet people, will you set aside a space for that purpose only?
   I will set aside an uncluttered space to meet people. ___yes___no
   If my answer is "no," how can I solve my need for a meeting space? _____
   _____
   _____.
8. Analyze why you have so many articles, booklets, and papers.
   Do I keep papers because I *think* I *ought* to keep them, but don't really know why I do it? _____yes
   Consider whether you are fearful you'll not be able to retrieve a piece of information in the future.
   I am fearful. _____yes
9. Instead of saving information for potential use, develop research skills. If you don't have research skills, would you like to learn a few research skills so you can use the Internet to acquire information you need at the time you need it? Then you don't have to be afraid you won't have what you need when you want it—and you can get rid of a lot of paper.
   I'd like to learn some basic research skills by taking a class or asking a friend to help me learn. _____yes

10. Some more things you can do.
    I am willing to simplify my life. _____yes
    I am willing to clean out anything I've not used in a year unless I have a specific plan for it at this time. _____yes

11. Consider obtaining the services of a professional organizer—but be careful the person knows about working with someone with an ADD style of brain construction. Otherwise, you'll never be able to implement the system the person has constructed for you. Interview the person. Be observant. Trust your feelings and answer the following:
    I'd like to try a professional organizer. _____yes
    The first thing I'll try to observe is whether I feel this person understands me. I feel the person _____does _____does not understand me.
    Do I feel twinges of guilt or discomfort or feelings of hopelessness as the person constructs an organizational system for me? _____yes
    If you answer "yes," you'll probably need to choose someone else.
    Is the person taking time to find out how I do things, how I think, and what I'm trying to accomplish? _____yes **This is a good sign.**
    Has a follow-up visit been planned to see if what has been planned actually will work for me? _____yes

Your Commitments:

I commit to follow through with the plans I've chosen. ___yes___no
I will begin to work on my first plan (insert date). _____
When I have made an effort to get my clutter under control, I will continue to work with my organizational skills in the following way and in the following time: _____
_____
_____ .

What Makes This Hard To Do:

There is a social value placed on neatness with a concomitant criticism of anyone who isn't neat. As a creative, active person, you will have to courageously stand up for the choices you make to work in a way that fits your particular style of brain construction.

SUBDUING STACKS AND PILES

Question:

Do you have trouble finding the floor in your home or space for your car because of the stacks and piles you've built?

Why This Happens:

- You are likely to have a broad vision—a big-picture perspective on the world that omits the details in your environment.
- You're probably very active and the thought of having to take the time to put each book or piece of paper in a particular place is more than you can stand.
- As a person who needs to tangibly see what you have to draw from, you've begun to organize in a way that fits your brainstyle. Kudos to you!
- You have likely taken on more than you can manage at one time or are trying to hang onto every little idea that crosses your path.
- You may be fearful that if you let go of anything—ideas, books, or dreams—they will be lost forever.
- You may be unsure of your path in life or not know how to achieve your dreams. As a result, you're trying to guarantee that you'll find what you're seeking.

Problems You Face Because of Stacks and Piles:

- Your committed other, roommate, or family may wish to "divorce you" because of your piles.
- You've tried to get rid of stuff, but even when you throw it away, the piles soon grow even higher.
- You feel ashamed.

Your Goal:

You want to make decisions and develop skills that will affect your stacks and piles permanently in such a way that you get what you want and others feel comfortable living or working around you.

What Not To Do:

Do not throw things out indiscriminately or give in to hopeless resignation.

Your Work:

1. If the stacks don't bother someone else, it's okay to leave them if you like.
   I will leave them. _____yes _____no
   I choose to eliminate them even though they don't bother anyone else. I will do this because _____
   _____ .

2. If you want to effectively change your habits, you must give yourself permission to make the change.
   I give myself permission to make changes to my stacks and piles. _____yes

3. If you hear a voice in your head saying stacks are bad and therefore it is bad for you to have them, tell your voice, "I am in control of my life. Thank you for making the suggestion, but I will do what I want."
   I want to say this. _____yes
   If the voice is insistent, get tough. Say, "Out of here. I don't need you. I'm in charge." Then get busy doing something you want to do, and forget trying to clear out your piles of stuff at this time.

4. To work on subduing your stacks and piles, consider calling upon a friend or acquaintance who can help you.
   I will call _____, _____,
   or _____.

5. Your helper can be your go-fer doing what you say is to be done.
   I will ask my helper to _____.

6. One way to proceed that often works well is to analyze your piles together. Your partner can pick up one item at a time. Then you say where it is to go. You can keep items or throw them away. Have three piles:
   Pile 1 will be a wastebasket or garbage bag for throwing things away.
   Pile 2 will contain items that are to be kept out in the open.
   Pile 3 will contain items that are to be stored.
   I agree to immediately throw away things I
      don't want or need.   _____yes
   I commit to only keep a half dozen or so
      books near me.   _____yes
   I will store the rest.   _____yes

7. If you want to keep several stacks of book, have your partner write labels or find attractive boxes or shelves to put them on once they've been arranged into categories such as "read now," "read later," "thumb through." Or you may arrange them by subject.
   I agree to do this. _____yes

8. If you buy books in order to hold onto a new interest or idea, reconsider.
   I agree to stop buying books just because I have a new idea or interest. _____yes

9. You don't *have* to act on every idea you have. Choose one idea at a time and stick with it. Send the other ideas back from whence they came. If they are important for you, they'll resurface to your consciousness again and again.
   I commit to work with one new idea at a time. _____yes

10. If you can't bear to part with an idea, write it down. There, you've saved it without adding to your stacks and piles.
    I can do this. _____yes

11. If you're searching for your identity or path in life by reading, go to the library to satisfy yourself rather than buying books.
    I commit to borrow books from friends or use the library rather than buy them so I can return them when I've finished with them. _____yes

12. If your stacks bother someone else, remind yourself that living with another person means you must take their wishes into account.
    Who in my life is bothered by my stacks and piles? _____
    I agree to work at reaching a consensus with the following people: _____, _____, _____ .

13. If you and your partner/roommate argue, each wanting control, seek relationship counseling.
    I am willing to seek relationship counseling whether the other person is willing to or not. _____yes
    Here is the name and phone number of at least one counselor with whom I can speak: _____

14. If your partner is good at organizing and you trust his or her judgment to be understanding of your needs, you may ask for help and even turn the organizing over to that person.

I have such a person in my life who I'd like to
consider using.   _____yes
Is the person willing to help me organize my
stacks and piles?   _____yes
If you answer "yes" to both questions, commit to turning
the job over.
I make the commitment to turn the job over to my partner.
_____yes

15. Whether you do the job yourself or you turn it over to
    someone else, work on only one area at a time.
    I commit to work on *one* area at a time.   _____yes

16. When you're finished with the one area, treat yourself and
    your partner to something you both enjoy.
    I agree to reward myself and my helper with _____
    _____ .

Your Commitments:

I commit to follow through with this plan.   _____yes
I commit to maintain this plan regularly.   _____yes

What Makes This Hard To Do:

Spending time organizing or reducing your stacks and piles is a
whole lot less pleasurable than acquiring them. But try fully savoring a few books and magazines at a time. Thoroughly read them.
Know you'll have time for more when you finish these.

CLEANING THE WHOLE HOUSE

Question:

Do your organizational skills defy your attempts to get big projects, such as cleaning the house, done?

Why This Happens:

- When you see the housecleaning project as *one* big project, it appears, and is, an *enormous* job.
- When you have a brainstyle that focuses on the big picture rather than on details, you are likely to have a problem knowing where to start to dissect a big project.
- The generally recommended systematic approach to tackling a big project rarely works for people with an ADD brainstyle.
- With a big-picture brainstyle, you are likely to be creative and therefore have a lot of different projects going at the same time. That's a lot of stuff to clean and organize.
- You are likely to prefer spending time with people or doing exciting, innovative things than cleaning house.
- The way you're taught you *should* clean house may not work for you.

Problems You Face Doing Big Projects:

- Though you would like to have a neat and orderly house, you seem incapable of achieving it.
- Every time you set aside time to clean it, you barely get started before you feel overwhelmed and give up.
- You get one or two things done and then get distracted.
- You may not get started at all because you have no idea where to start.

Your Goal:

You want to be able to get big projects such as housecleaning under your control.

What Not To Do:

Do not try to clean your house all at once or use an approach that doesn't fit your style of brain construction.

Your Work:

1. Be clear about your motivations and know you have choices about making the project *your* goal and how you go about it. Some people find things just fine in cluttered settings.
   I agree to seek the following ways:

   _____

   _____ .

2. How you go about achieving your goal means you must use your brainstyle to advantage. Start by looking at the function served by the project. In the case of housecleaning, ask yourself what the function of a clean house is for you.
   Do I want to be neat so someone will stop
      nagging me?   _____yes
   Do I want to be neat to please another person
   or because I think I *should*?   _____yes
   Do I choose to clean house (or complete a
      big project) because I want the end result?   _____yes
3. Once you've committed, it's important to break your house-cleaning or any project into manageable portions and find a style of cleaning that fits you.
   I commit to break my housecleaning projects
      into manageable portions.   _____yes
   I commit to find my own style of accomplishing
      the task.   _____yes
4. It may help you to think of housecleaning as a *process*, not a one-time job.
   When I think of housecleaning as a process, this is what I think it will look like to me: _____
5. Now it's time to become more specific. Ask yourself:
   Am I willing to start on my cleaning job? _____yes
   If you are, here are some of the areas to consider:
   How much time am I willing to spend when I work on the project? _____
   How many rooms or parts of rooms am I willing to clean at a time? _____
   How neat or thoroughly do I want to clean?
   _____a little _____moderately _____a lot _____perfectly
   Let your feelings be your guide. If you choose "perfectly," ask yourself why you need that standard. Ask yourself:
   Did I learn it?   _____yes
   Am I driven in everything I do to be perfect?   _____yes

If your answer is "yes," you could be facing a challenge with what is called "obsessive-compulsive disorder." Consider consulting a professional (psychiatrist, physician, or psychologist) for help. This is not a condition of "will," but is a biochemical issue.

6. Next choose which of two cleaning styles you'd like to try out to do your cleaning.

    Style 1. You work with an entire space, moving through it as an improvisational dancer might move through space. For example, you move clothes left in the living room to the bedroom closet. On the floor by the side of the bed, you see some things that need to go to the bathroom, so you swoop down, pick them up, and dance to the bathroom. There, you stop and clean the sink and tub before gathering up what needs to be washed. Then, off you go to put in a load of wash. This works if you see the overall big picture in your mind and have lots of energy to burn off.

    Style 2. You choose one small area and clear it completely. This could be only one-fourth of a tabletop.

    You may try first one style and then the other. Ask yourself:
    Which one do I want to try first? _____ Style 1 _____ Style 2
    When you've finished your trials, which one do you like best?
    I prefer _____ Style 1 _____ Style 2 _____ both

7. Regardless of which style you choose, you need to create three piles. You can use garbage bags or boxes for the following piles:

    Pile 1. Label this pile, "Throw away."
    Pile 2. Label this pile, "I can't live without this."
    Pile 3. Label this pile, "I don't know."

    Put the "I don't know" pile away for six months or a year and then go through it again. Immediately throw away the "Throw away" pile. Take time to decide where to put the things that you can't live without.
    I want to try the three pile methods of dealing with items.
    _____ yes

8. If you become overwhelmed doing your big project, you may be trying to do too much or for too long. Break your work into smaller bits.
    Do I agree to do this? _____ yes

9. Carefully choose the places you want to put what you keep. Open shelves and flat surfaces may work well for people who have problems with "out of sight, out of mind."

Would you like to try using shelves and flat surfaces to store things? _____yes _____no
If not, what would you like to substitute?
I would like to store things in or on _____
_____ .

10. To better keep your house or work area straight, have out-of-the-way places to do your creative, inventive projects that you only clean up *after* you finish a project. Do not let anyone else get into those areas.
    If you agree with this idea, write: "I think this it is a good idea to have out-of-the-way places to do my creative, inventive projects."

    _____

    _____

11. Do you like to spend time with people? _____yes _____no
    If you do, have someone around to keep you company even if they don't help you with the cleaning. It will boost your motivation.
    People I will ask to keep me company while I work with this big project are _____ and

    _____

Your Commitments:

I will commit to try various methods for tackling a   _____yes
  big project such as house cleaning.   _____no
I plan to begin work on my plan (insert date): _____
    After you've implemented your plan, evaluate your satisfaction with your progress.

_____

_____

What Makes This Hard To Do:

It takes time to discover a system that works for you. And finding the right one is complex. So first work on your motives, the style you wish to follow, and then practice it, training yourself over time.

KEEPING TRACK OF PERSONAL FINANCES

Question:

Do you find you're continually having trouble keeping up with bills and financial information?

Why This Happens:

- Keeping track of bills and receipts is a very linear, detailed job—one that does not use the skills that may make up your strengths.
- If you are a big-picture person who sees the overview of situations and automatically pays attention to how things function or are used, you may be able to recall a picture of when and why you generated the bills and receipts, but not actually find them.
- The individual bits of paper are not a part of your perceptual world.

Problems You Face Keeping Up With Bills and Financial Information:

- You don't pay bills you need to pay.
- You don't have any idea where the receipt is to return something to a store.
- You have no idea where to find what you need in order to file your income tax, much less what to do about the other years you haven't filed even though you meant to.
- Your family is threatened with overwhelming debt.
- A primary relationship is about to end because of your difficulties managing finances.

Your Goal:

To get your finances under control so you don't live in crisis and can find an organizational system that fits you.

What Not To Do:

Don't do "nothing." But also, don't beat up on yourself.

Your Work:

1. You must come face-to-face with your situation, admitting that you're out of control with a task that your Accommodating You must find a solution to while avoiding further wounding to your True Self.
   It's time for me to face my financial problems.
   I will do it.   _____yes
2. You need to agree to commit to an overhaul of your financial management habits.
   I am willing to commit to an overhaul.   _____yes
3. Immediately deal with the IRS. If you feel intimidated, be sure to get the help of either a professional, a financial service, or someone you know who is extremely knowledgeable about such things.
   I will use one of the following resources: _____ or
   _____ .
4. You must ask for help to get your other financial problems under control. This can be a credit counseling service, a bookkeeper or accountant, or a friend or relative.
   I will begin by asking the following people to help me:
   _____ , _____ , or
   _____ .
5. Seriously consider cutting up your credit cards.
   I know I need to do this. _____yes, and I will do it.   _____yes
6. Some people do better with debit cards while others need to tangibly see what they are doing with their transactions.
   I want to try a debit arrangement.   _____yes
   I like using a debit card.   _____yes
   I want to use a combination of cash and
      checks for my spending.   _____yes
   I like using cash and checks.   _____yes
   Some people need to go to an all-cash system to get and keep control of their spending. You can keep your cash in envelopes for various categories of spending, such as food, gas, utilities, and discretionary spending.
   I want to try using cash only. _____yes
7. After the crisis is over, you must work on an organizational system that fits you, so you never again have to become desperate.
   I also will follow through to get a system that will work in the future. _____yes

8. Today is a new day and the past is the past. This means you must not let your feeling of remorse immobilize you or keep you from acting to solve your problem now.
Even though I feel bad about my financial mess, I am willing to resist feeling ashamed. _____yes

9. *If you once had a system that worked for you,* even some of the time, recall when and why you stopped using it. Write down your story.

_____

_____

10. How did my previous system work?

_____

_____

11. What has helped you gain financial order in the past? Check the ways that have worked for you.
A special place to put your bills and receipts _____yes
Use of colored folders to help you keep track
    of your financial papers _____yes
Stacking financial matters that need telephone
    intervention next to your phone _____yes
Placing computer related matters next to
    your computer _____yes
A special place to collect what you need to take
    to your bookkeeper or accountant for your
    income tax or other accounting needs _____yes
Making a list of things to do in a timely manner _____yes
Using a computer program to enter
    financial matters _____yes
Using a debit card system _____yes
I will commit to use whatever ways were
    effective previously. _____yes
Will you set small, achievable goals and congratulate yourself every time you reach one?

_____

_____

12. *If you have no history with a system that worked for you,* it's time to find one—a system or person who can help you develop something that will help you manage your personal finances. The system or person must be sensitive to your style of brain construction so that they come up with help

that you can utilize. The best way for you to tell if you've found the right person for you is whether you follow what the person is doing and see if it feels comfortable.

I will consider a new system and carefully choose one that fits my brainstyle. _____yes

13. Be willing to try several approaches.
I am willing to try several approaches. _____yes

14. Try any of the ways outlined under #11 that appeal to you.
After trying the different ways, I find I like

_____

_____ .

Also try doing your bill paying and bank reconciliations at the same place and time.
I like this idea. _____yes
Choose a place where you can relax such as out-of-doors, in bed, or _____ .
I feel I'd like to try the following places._____ .
Reward yourself when you pay bills, saying "thank you" for the use of the products or services that the money paid for. Choose a specific reward when you reconcile your bank statement.
I will reward myself by or with _____ .

15. As you discover or think up new approaches to managing your finances, fill in the following information.
Approach 1. Description: _____

_____
Date started _____ I was comfortable—uncomfortable (circle one) using it.
Approach 2. Description _____

_____
Date started _____ I was comfortable—uncomfortable (circle one) using it.
Approach 3. Description _____

_____
Date started _____ I was comfortable—uncomfortable (circle one) using it.

16. You may wish to consider hiring or making a trade with someone to *permanently* manage the personal or business finances in your life.
Would you like to hire someone or make a trade? _____yes

I will talk to _____ about taking
over my finances indefinitely.
I will trade the following, if possible:

_____ .

Your Commitments:

I commit to finding a system that will work for me. _____yes
I commit to regain control immediately if my system
   breaks down in the future. _____yes

What Makes This Hard To Do:

Your style of brain construction can make dealing with your personal finances next to impossible. The feelings of shame and guilt that result tend to make you hide from them. Being overwhelmed keeps you from making headway in dealing with them. Not knowing where to start gets in the way.

The problem is that the IRS and bill collectors won't go away. So face the music sooner rather than later. You may not be talented in handling paperwork, but you are not a bad person because you're having trouble. Ask for help to accommodate to a job that doesn't fit the way you're made.

MANAGING PAPER AT WORK

Question:

Do you do wonderfully on your job except for the paperwork?

Why This Happens:

- You are being called upon to do two or more totally different jobs under the label of one.
- Each job requires you to use different areas of your brain. The area that manages accounting and keeps track of details is different from the part that makes you so talented and skillful in the important areas of your job—the areas you like.
- Rarely, if ever, are people equally good at both sets of skills.

Problems You Face Managing Paperwork:

- You are skillful at all aspects of your job except keeping track of what you've accomplished.
- Tracking expenditures, sales, profits, time, mileage, and even income may be beyond you.
- You may jeopardize losing a job you like because of your inability to manage paperwork.
- You may end up shortchanged because you don't submit the paperwork needed to get paid.
- A family member may suffer or get angry at you.

Your Goal:

To find a way to manage your paperwork/bookkeeping on the job—one that you can maintain over time.

What Not To Do:

Do not expect yourself to necessarily be good at everything on the job. But don't avoid the parts that are hard. They will catch up with you sooner or later.

Your Work:

1. To be effective in learning to manage your paperwork and bookkeeping on the job, you need to commit to changing your ways so you find a system that works for you.

I agree to spend time seeking a system that fits my brain-style. _____yes _____ no
If you answer "no," what do you want to do instead?
Instead, I will _____

_____ .

2. To begin work on getting your paperwork under control, you need to recognize that you don't do everything equally well.
   I acknowledge that I don't do everything equally well. I have both strengths and weaknesses. _____yes

3. You must be willing to spend more time utilizing your strengths than wasting time on what you don't do well.

4. You may have a lot of negative thoughts running through your mind that will distract you from getting your paperwork done.
   I am willing to argue with my negative thoughts. _____ yes
   You might say to your thoughts, "I can find a way that fits me, so go away ugly thoughts."

5. Make a list of what you do and don't do well so you can make trades with someone else to do what you don't do well.

What I do well	What I don't do well
_____	Paperwork _____
_____	_____
_____	_____

6. Notice similarities between the items in list 1 and those in the items in list 2.
   I see the following similarities in the items in list 1: _____

   _____

   _____ .

   I see the following similarities in the items in list 2: _____

   _____

   _____ .

7. One way around your problems with paperwork is to look for someone on the job who can do the tasks that are hard for you.
   Immediately, I think of _____ or _____ .
   What can you trade with that person to make it worth his or her while to help you?
   The person's name

   _____

   _____

What I can trade

_____

_____

8. If you can't find someone to help, talk to your boss about having a person assigned to keep track of your clerical work. Point out that you'll bring in more business or create more product because of the help you receive. The clerical help will end up paying for itself.
   I'd like to do this. _____yes

9. If you have to do the job yourself, go easy on yourself so you don't waste energy on self-blame.
   I agree to do the job myself without wasting time or energy being self-critical. _____yes

10. Begin by determining how you best work. Are you the kind of person who does better doing a little bit of something hard and then taking a break?
    When I think about how I prefer to work, I do like to break projects into pieces, doing a little, then taking a break, then doing some more. _____yes

11. If you answer "yes," then deal with your paperwork daily or even immediately after every sale or accomplishment.
    Am I willing to try this? _____yes
    I will deal with my paperwork: _____ daily _____ after each step.

12. Set yourself up to do your paperwork in an environment that fits you. Which of the following pleases you?
    The out-of-doors   _____yes   _____no
    A quiet setting   _____yes   _____no
    Around others   _____yes   _____no
    At home   _____yes   _____no
    With music, radio, or TV _____yes   _____no
    Some other environment _____

13. Giving yourself a reward when you're done often helps people do what is hard or unpleasant.
    I will reward myself with _____ .

14. Some people would rather do their organizational work all at once rather than in bits and pieces, so they don't lose their train of thought. If you like the all-at-once method, you will need to determine how often you want to do your paperwork.
    I would like to try doing my paperwork:
    Weekly   _____yes _____no

Monthly   _____yes _____no
Quarterly   _____yes _____no
Other   _____

15. After several tries that fail, do not delude yourself into thinking that you can do the job *the next time.*
    I have tried several times to do my paperwork by myself and it's not working. _____yes

16. If you answer "yes" to this question, it's time to get help. Either return to your boss, ask a coworker, or consider asking someone outside the job. You may want or need to pay this person, but that's okay if you like the job enough to stay with it.
    I will ask _____ or _____ .
    My relation to that person suggests I need to offer to pay him or her. _____yes

17. Finally, if you can't find a solution to successfully do the amount of paperwork your job demands, or you don't want to keep having to do it, you need to change jobs. Don't wait to be fired and don't compromise your mental health.
    I plan to begin to look for a job that utilizes my strengths and requires me to use my weaknesses less of the time. _____yes

Your Commitments:

I commit to start managing my paperwork (date): _____
I also commit to check my system regularly.   _____yes
If you get behind in the future, you must immediately set aside time to remedy your lapse and look at your plan again to see where it needs modification.
I commit to immediately attend to any lapse in
  keeping up with my paperwork.   _____yes

What Makes This Hard To Do:

Although people who are usually good at clerical work are not expected to be creative or particularly expressive or mechanical, everyone is expected to be able to do clerical work. You are not allowed to say, "I'm not talented at clerical work," whereas others may say, "I'm not musically, artistically, or mechanically talented."

WRITING A REPORT

Question:

Do you spend way too much time organizing a report and still not do a very good job?

Why This Happens:
- As someone who *feels* your way through a writing task, or any project for that matter, you are not likely to be able to begin at the beginning.
- You probably don't think or write in little steps.
- You are likely, when you begin a task like this, to have information and ideas churning around in your mind with no beginning, middle, or end in sight.

Problems You Face Writing a Report:
- You spend too much time trying to get organized.
- You experience too much stress and dread tackling the job.
- You get frustrated trying to write an outline ahead of time and it actually slows you down.
- You're pretty sure your end result isn't very good.

Your Goal:

Learn to write a report or document without having to expend undue energy. If it is a report that you write repetitively, construct a template that will make your job easier.

What Not To Do:

Do not give up because you feel you'll never be able to produce a worthwhile report.

Your Work:
1. The main reason for difficulty, even failure, to write a report is because you've been trying to go about writing it in a way that doesn't fit your brainstyle. Are you willing to try one

more time, this time using methods that are more likely to fit your brainstyle?

I am willing to try again using methods that will probably better fit me. _____yes _____no

If you've answered "no," what do you want to do about your report writing?

I propose that I do the following in relation to my report writing: _____
_____ .

2. Are you willing to set aside the ways you've previously been taught that haven't worked for you?

   I agree to set ways aside that haven't worked for me before. _____yes

3. Changing the order in which you write the report is one way to improve your efficiency. Are you willing to progress through the writing of the report in a different order from the eventual order of the report? For example, you may leave the introduction until the end to write. You may start with a midsection of the report that is easy for you to produce.

   I will try a new way of ordering the writing of my report. _____yes

4. You must first be clear about the parameters of the report you are planning to write. Answer the following questions so you understand the limits and intent of your report.

   Who is the report being written for? _____

   What is the purpose of the report? _____

   What does the report need to contain to be complete? _____
   _____

   Will you need to do the same kind of report (project) repeatedly? _____yes

5. Next, brainstorm.

   Would you prefer to brainstorm alone?   _____yes

   With someone else?   _____yes

   With a group?   _____yes

6. To brainstorm, use a piece of paper or a white board, write down as many components of the report as you can. Anything you think of that's related to the report gets written at this time. This could include an introduction, background,

conclusions, summary, explanation of new events since the last report, effects of the new events, key players, and so on.

Use single words or short phrases. Draw pictures. Do not necessarily make a list, though that's okay. Brainstorm below:

_____

_____

_____

_____

_____

_____

_____

_____

_____

_____

_____

_____

7. You can also begin organizing your report by putting each idea related to the project down on a card and lay the cards on a table or the floor to arrange them.
   I am willing to try this method. _____yes

8. Take a break after your brainstorming. Then step back from the words and pictures you've accumulated. This way you can scan the page. This approach fits a big-picture brain-style. You'll begin to *feel* what goes together.
   I commit to try working this way. _____yes

9. Notice what subjects and words draw your attention repeatedly. This is likely to lead to the place for you to start writing your report.
   I see that I am drawn to the following subjects and words:

   _____

   _____ .

10. If you notice two words together, even though they're separated in space on the paper, that may mean they belong together in the report.
    I pair up the following words as I look at the paper: _____

    _____ .

11. List the categories of items that begin to emerge. Then place these categories into several major groups, making fewer, but larger categories. With this you are beginning to create clusters.

_____
_____
_____
_____
_____
_____
_____
_____
_____
_____
_____
_____

12. One cluster will seem to precede another cluster as the report starts to take shape. Feel your way along. List these
clusters in the order you feel they belong.

_____
_____
_____
_____
_____
_____
_____
_____
_____
_____
_____

13. Decide which section to work on next. Remember, you
don't need to start at the beginning. Let your feelings guide
you.
I feel I would like to begin with _____ .

14. You may also find it's more effective for you to work on the
whole project a little at a time rather than working on one section and honing it to completion before turning to the next.
I would prefer to work a little at a time on the whole project.
_____yes

15. After you've worked on most of the sections of the report
and have them in an order you are fairly pleased with, it's
time to look at the whole report from beginning to end. A
big-picture person makes several run throughs of the whole

report—one run through for content, one to be sure the sections are connected the way you want them, another for editing, and so on.

I would like to try working this way. I'll ignore details but start by seeing if the report seems to be coming together in a way that makes sense to me. _____yes

16. During the writing of the report and certainly after you've finished, let what you've written sit for a time. When you come back to it, you'll more clearly see what you want to change.

    I agree to try this. _____yes

17. If you have to write a similar document in the future, outline the paper *after* it is finished. Then you can use the same outline time after time.

    I agree to make an outline that I can keep for the future. _____yes

18. If you really feel lost after you've tried these suggestions, don't hesitate to ask someone to help you. Or even if you're making headway with your report writing, you may still wish to contact an editor to edit your work or work alongside you while you're writing. Be sure, however, that the person is sensitive to your brainstyle.

    Often working beside an editor on a document teaches you, kinesthetically, how to write a document yourself. It may take a couple of times working this way, but it can create marvelous results.

    I would like to seek help. _____yes
    I will ask _____.
    If you try someone and start feeling anxious, overwhelmed, or emotional, you may need to try someone else. Though it may take time, you'll find the right person. Trust your response. The problem is not you. It's only a problem of fit between the editor and the writer.

Your Commitments:

I am willing to realize that my difficulty writing reports has always had less to do with my innate skills and more to do with the way in which I was taught to do them. I know this was no one's fault.   _____yes

I commit to be kind to myself allowing my report
   writing skills to emerge slowly.   _____yes
I commit to seek writing help if I need it.   _____yes

What Makes This Hard To Do:

Your worst enemy may be your feelings. Feeling overwhelmed with
no idea of where to start can block your progress. Thinking you
ought to start at the beginning and work sequentially through to
the end may stall your progress.

Be sure to breathe and use your inner feelings to see what you're
drawn to do, one step at a time, no matter what your order of writing.

PUTTING OFF STARTING THINGS

Question:

Do you procrastinate starting projects?

Why This Happens:

- Starting things early may not fit your brainstyle even though there's a *belief* that one ought to do a little bit at a time spread over regular intervals.
- You may naturally work better when you wait until a deadline is close.
- Big-picture people often have to work a project out in their mind, outside of conscious awareness, before being able to begin the project and work with details of the project.
- We all have our own rhythm for working and doing. Many spontaneous, creative people get an assignment, check out the parameters of it, and then tuck the assignment in the back of their minds. Several days may go by before they actually *begin* the project.
- If you are a creative, big-picture person, your project may come out in one big whole with little editing or detail work necessary.

Problems You Face Because of Procrastination:

- You fail to get around to starting a project that has a due date.
- You gain a reputation of being irresponsible and of putting things off.
- Even though you get your work done at the last minute, you're nagged or criticized about getting it done in a more timely manner. You don't know how to do that.

Your Goal:

To feel good about the way you naturally accomplish goals and deadlines in a timely manner.

What Not To Do:

Do not get down on yourself because you put things off to the last minute. Do not try to fit a production schedule that's not made for your particular style of brain construction.

Your Work:

1. To begin to handle the timing of starting a project, you must be truly willing to do what you've committed to do.
   I will be sure that I only commit to projects that I am willing to do. _____yes

2. To successfully complete projects, you must give yourself permission to work on a project in your own way in your own time.
   I will set the parameters of when and how I'll work on a project. _____yes

3. Often people don't trust themselves because they've been told repeatedly that the way they approach a project is not right. Has this happened to you?
   I was told I didn't do things in the right way or the right time. _____yes

4. Yet you can be effective and acceptable when you do projects in your own way in your own time.
   I am willing to change my thinking to know that I can do things in my own way. _____yes

5. As you learn about a project, be certain you understand the parameters of the assignment. Think of an assignment you have pending and answer the following questions:
   Who am I doing the project for? _____
   What do I need to get across in it? _____
   _____
   How long does it need to be? _____
   How long do I estimate it will take me to do it if I do it all at once?
   _____
   _____.

6. Using a month-at-a-glance calendar can be very useful in getting a handle on how long a project will take. It is a visual way to figure your timing on your project. The first few times you use this scheme you may find your timing is a bit off. But you'll adjust as you gain practice until you pretty much get your timing down. Fill in the following dates.
   My project is due _____. I will mark that date on my calendar.
   Next, I'll subtract one or two days for miscellaneous problems like running into a computer glitch. I will then mark this date on my calendar.

I will then ask myself how long I would like to spend working on the actual construction of the whole project. _____ I'll subtract this time.

Now you'll know when you'll probably need to begin the actual production.

7. After the general layout of your timing, you need to make special preparations to begin the project such as ordering materials, renting equipment, interviewing people, networking with colleagues, and so on.

    I need to make the following special preparations in order to begin my project: _____

    _____ .

8. What materials do you need to order? _____

    _____

9. Who do you need to interview or network with? _____

    _____

10. What research is there for you to do? _____

    _____

    Mark your calendar in relation to the special preparations you need to make. When do you want to make the preparations you need to make?

    I need to make them _____ .

11. Once you've set the parameters of the project down and completed planning for the special preparations you need to make, you can put the project in the back of your mind and let your creative mind flush it out.

12. Begin the actual writing or production when you *feel* it is the right time to start. This may be the time you previously marked down to start the project or it may even be earlier. Compare the time you estimated earlier with your current feeling of whether it is the *right* time for you to begin.

    When I compare the planned starting time and my current starting time, how close was my estimation? _____days

13. If your planned starting time is different from your current timing, listen carefully to your feelings *and* think about the discrepancy, then readjust your work schedule.

    My new work schedule is _____

    _____ .

14. When it's time for you to begin work, review the parameters—who, what, and how. Close your eyes, take a deep breath, and

ask your creative self to begin the process of creating the project. Within seconds, a picture, word, or thought will jump into your mind. With that, you're off and running.

Here's what came to my mind: _____

_____

_____ .

15. If you're criticized for your style, simply tell people you have the situation under control and that you'll take responsibility for completing the project in a timely manner. Write what you'll say to those who criticize or question you.

_____

_____

_____

Your Commitments:

I commit to be responsible to my way of doing things.   _____yes

I will be polite, but resist others' attempts to criticize   _____yes
   or judge the way I do things.

I am willing to be responsible for things that I undertake. _____yes

What Makes This Hard To Do:

Changing a belief about yourself and the way in which you work is hard. You'll have to convince yourself that it's okay to do assignments in your own way.

TALKING OFF TRACK

Question:

Do you get off track when you are talking?

Why This Happens:

- As a person whose brain focuses on the patterns, interconnections, and relationships between things more than on specific bits of information, you are likely to drift away from one thought to a complex of thoughts.
- The True You is a big-picture person who tends to tell stories and describe whole scenes to make your point when you're speaking. On your goal path, you see something to the side of the path that will enrich your description, even make it more understandable. You share it and get off the main track you've been on.
- You tend to get totally immersed in what you're doing—living it as you are speaking about it. This makes you forget a pre-planned outline or objective goal path.
- You are likely to experience shame over "losing your train of thought." Then, feeling shame, you are likely to become further distracted as you pay attention to your feelings.

Problems You Face Because of Talking Off Track:

- You feel bad because not everyone in the audience appreciates the way you present.
- The biggest problem isn't that you get off track, but that you can't remember what you were saying before you took the mental side trip while you were speaking.
- You feel ashamed, "bad," or inadequate because you get off track.
- Others may think you are disorganized, unprofessional, irresponsible, or a poor presenter who doesn't know your subject.

Your Goal:

To learn to anchor your initial thought while enriching your speaking with side trips.

What Not To Do:

Do not let yourself feel helplessly lost from your original path.

Your Work:

1. People with a brainstyle similar to yours will more than likely appreciate the way in which you make presentations. Those with a different brainstyle will probably be uncomfortable or stressed or have trouble understanding you.
   I realize that my way of speaking is valid for people with a brainstyle similar to mine. They will often learn effectively from my stories and side trips. _____yes

2. All brainstyles will be in the audiences to which you present. You need to make an effort to reach a wide range of brainstyles.
   I want to make every effort to reach a wide range of brainstyles with my presentations. _____yes

3. When you tell a story or take a side trip during a presentation, you will need to be able to return to your central theme. The key is to make a *purposeful* decision to take a side trip instead of just letting it happen to you. You do this by engaging your left brain and stating either to yourself or your audience what you are planning to do.
   I will purposely decide when I want to make a side trip during a presentation. _____yes

4. You must "anchor" the point at which you get off your path. Anchoring makes it easier to return to your original point when you've finished your side trip. To anchor your decision to make a side trip, you can verbalize that decision to the person to whom you're speaking, to someone in your audience, or to a physical place in the near environment. You also want to say it to yourself.
   I will anchor my decision when I choose to make a side trip. _____yes

5. Note where you are placing your anchor with a gesture, such as pointing your finger downward as if you were casting an anchor into the water or pointing your finger toward a person in the audience. You may want to keep your hand in that position all the time you are telling your story.
   I will practice making this or another gesture of my choosing the next time I'm talking to a group. _____yes

6. If you are speaking to another person, you can anchor where you leave the main path by touching the other's arm. You may want to hold that position until you are finished with your example.
   I will experiment with ways to stay anchored during a one-on-one conversation. _____yes
   Some ways that I can think of trying are: _____
   _____.

7. When you are talking to a group, you can ask someone in the audience to remember where you leave the verbal path. Ironically, having asked, you are likely to remember yourself. And audience members often feel more involved in what you're talking about because of their participation in your presentation.
   The next time I make a presentation to a group I am willing to ask someone to help me anchor where I leave the main path during my presentation. _____yes

Your Commitments:

I commit to try various anchoring techniques.   _____yes
I commit to value my way of presenting and will
   make an effort to make it reach a wide audience.   _____yes

What Makes This Hard To Do:

Embarrassment and fear that you won't be able to overcome getting off track is likely to make it hard for you to change. Perhaps you think you shouldn't need to do anything to stay on track. These fears often make us feel helpless to change our situation. Just remember, you are not helpless.

GETTING PLACES ON TIME

Question:

Do you run the risk of not getting important places on time?

Why This Happens:

- Intending to leave early enough to get somewhere on time does not mean you know how to do it.
- Figuring out the amount of time you need to accomplish a task can be very difficult for those people with a large number of ADD attributes.
- "Telling time" by a clock, especially a digital clock, and "keeping time" are linear activities involving *unnatural* measurements such as minutes and hours. This is in opposition to telling time by using the natural rhythms of nature, such as watching the sun or using your own body's rhythms.
- If you are untrained to be in touch with your natural environment, you may think you have more time than you actually do to get somewhere.
- Often the suggestion is made to simply add fifteen or thirty minutes to the time you would normally leave to go somewhere. People with a nonlinear brainstyle are likely to fill in that *extra* time with all kinds of additional activities and be even later than they would have without the extra time.
- Being an active person, you tend to get involved in lots of activities at the same time, including doing things that have nothing to do with getting to your destination on time.

Problems You Face Because You Have Trouble Getting Places On Time:

- You miss or are late for important engagements both in your personal life and your work world.
- Those who count on you are affected by your trouble with time, nag you, or get angry at you.
- You feel ashamed and guilty because you keep failing.

Your Goal:

To get places on time or accept the repercussions of failing to do so without putting someone else at jeopardy.

What Not To Do:

Do not ignore the problem, compounding your guilt and jeopardizing your job or a relationship.

Your Work:

1. To effectively get your timing under control in a way that will work for your natural self, you must believe you can do it.
    I believe I can accomplish this with new methods. _____yes _____no
    If you answer "no," why do you fear you won't succeed?
    I am afraid I won't be able to succeed because _____
    _____ .

2. Learning new ways to think about time and timing can help you succeed. Are you willing to try?
    I am willing to try even though it feels scary. _____yes

3. The use of an analog clock instead of a digital clock is the first step. Identify the types of clocks you have in your life such as a wristwatch, those in your house, office, car, or computer. Notice whether they are analog or digital.
    I have _____ analog clocks and _____ digital clocks in my life.

4. Look at an analog clock. You will quickly note the time by where the clock's minute hand is in the pattern of the circle (pie). Is the minute hand close to the top of the circle at the 12 o'clock position, near the 3 o'clock position, at the bottom of the circle near the 6 o'clock position, or around the 9 o'clock position? These estimates will give you a clear *feeling* for what time it is. You don't have to be exact, but rather your sense of time will be stimulated by the proximity of the clock hand to a particular part of the circle (pie). As a big-picture person, this will have meaning for you, registering on your awareness.
    As I look at an analog clock, I realize I can "read the pattern" created by the position of the hands and I more easily know what time it is. _____yes

5. To make use of your particular brainstyle, break up the time it takes you to get to your destination.
    I am willing to try this in relation to a common destination to which I travel. _____yes

6. Begin by working backward from your destination. Don't use exact times. Rather, round all numbers up to the next quarter

hour of time. For example, if it will take you twenty-five minutes to leave your house, write down thirty minutes. If getting gas is likely to take eight minutes, write down fifteen minutes.

I will do this. _____ yes

7. Next, ask yourself the following questions:

What destination do I want to work with? _____

What time do I need to arrive at my destination? _____

I'll consider what I need to do in order to drive my vehicle from my home or office to the destination. _____ yes

How long will it take me to prepare to leave? For example, from home this may include getting the kids ready to go out the door or loading suitcases into the car. _____

How long will it take me to drive to my destination? _____

I'll add extra time if it's during rush hour. _____

I'll add extra time if I have to stop for errands on my way to my destination. This includes getting gas, dropping the kids off at school, or picking up my dry cleaning. _____

Next I'll add the numbers together, and I'll have the time I need between leaving my residence and arriving at my destination.

8. Post the time it takes on your calendar, on your refrigerator, or another visible place. This will serve as a reminder until you become habituated to the time it takes to get to the particular destination with which you've chosen to work.

I will post my timetable on _____ .

9. If you characteristically keep your spouse or coworker waiting, tell that person to go on ahead. If you're not ready, under no circumstances should that person wait for you. That would be enabling you to stay irresponsible about time.

Are you willing to be tough with yourself when someone else is involved? _____ yes

10. Who do you have in your life that you keep waiting so that they are late?

I jeopardize the following people at home and work: _____
_____ .

11. You must speak about your lateness to that person today and ask him or her to leave without you no matter what.

I agree to do this. _____ yes

12. If you continue to allow someone to enable your lateness, consider that one of you has a deeper psychological problem

than that created by an ADD brainstyle. This requires relationship counseling to solve.

I realize that we have a relationship problem
    that needs counseling.   _____yes

I am willing to get assistance, at least for myself. _____yes

13. A tip for those who fear getting somewhere early and being bored: take something to read or something to do in case you get to your destination early.

    I can take _____.

Your Commitments:

I commit to congratulate myself for taking charge of
   my time.   _____yes

If I slip in the future and begin to hold up people,
   or if others allow me to get sloppy, I will
   immediately refigure my timetable, implement it,
   or pay for the repercussions of being out of control. _____yes

What Makes This Hard To Do:

The biggest problem comes when someone takes responsibility for your timing while you are learning. You must be certain that no one is waiting on you. That person is shortchanging you, robbing you of your ability to learn to be responsible. You may have to be very emphatic with someone who unwittingly sabotages your progress this way.

Another hindrance comes from someone nagging you "to get going." The natural reaction is to move even slower in opposition to the nagging. Simply say, "You're not helping. I'd appreciate your backing off. I'll take care of things."

What also makes time management hard is that you are dealing with a habit that may be long-standing and habits are always hard to break. But you can do it.

REFUELING YOUR ENERGY

Question:

Do you have trouble organizing your eating and sleeping habits?

Why This Happens:

- As a baby, you may have had trouble settling into a *regular* schedule. Sensitive infants can have a tough time settling into the world of booming, buzzing, clattering confusion that prevails in most households, especially those with multitasking parents, so you never develop energy-restoring habits.
- You have your own internal time clock. Today's work favors day people and puts a great burden on those who do well at night.
- If you have a lot of sensitivity to stimuli that distract you from your work, you may prefer nighttime for working because it is quiet.
- When you don't naturally fit the demands of the timetable that defines your life, you are likely to need energy boosters to keep going, such as coffee and chocolate.
- Eating regularly means you must make the time to do that, which also means you will be on a regular schedule. But if you are a "go with the flow" type of person, you probably don't live on a regular schedule and don't much want to.
- Nutritious means are not easily available on fast-food row. It takes planning to get fresh produce and meat or grow your own. The complexities of preparing food from scratch may seem too much for you to face.

Problems You Face Because You Have Trouble Organizing Your Self-Care Habits:

- You may fail to get good nutrition because you skip meals or grab caffeinated drinks and junk food.
- You may have a hard time getting to sleep and a hard time waking up.
- You may feel tired all the time.
- Your health and efficiency may suffer.

Your Goal:

To find a natural eating and sleeping schedule that fits you.

What Not To Do:

Do not give up on the idea of eating nutritiously and getting satisfactory sleep.

Your Work:

1. To keep your energy level up and your health in good shape, it is important that you eat and sleep in ways that fit you.
   I want to go on a campaign to find nutritious but easy ways to obtain food that I like. _____yes
   I will spend the next month seeking a way to get these foods easily so that I don't have to make a continual *effort* to eat regularly and nutritiously. _____yes

2. If you like to *study* things in depth, systematically check out different foods you like and stick to them. Just be sure there is a balance of protein foods, fresh greens and vegetables, fruits, and some treats. Add dairy products if your body tolerates them. Make a list as you make your choices.

Protein	Vegetables	Fruits	Treats	Dairy
_____	_____	_____	_____	_____
_____	_____	_____	_____	_____
_____	_____	_____	_____	_____

3. If you don't like to systematically approach your planning, make a list of foods you like and add acceptable items that are missing. Keep the number of foods relatively small so you don't get overwhelmed with too many choices.
   My favorite foods include: _____
   _____
   _____ .
   Additional foods I'm willing to consider: _____
   _____
   _____ .

4. Seasonally change the foods you include. By tuning into your body's natural desires, you'll find that they tend to follow the

seasons of the year with hot, heavier foods in the winter and lighter foods in the summer.

What season of the year is it now? _____

What foods am I drawn to at this time? _____

_____

5. Decide if you want to eat out or at home most of the time.

I prefer to _____eat out _____eat at home.

6. If you prefer to eat out, choose places that serve "healthy" food. You may be surprised how adaptive many cooks and chefs are these days. Let them know what you want. Remember, you can take your food to go if you're "on the run."

Here are five places that are convenient where I can get food that will fit my healthy living style: _____,

_____, _____,

_____, and _____ .

7. You may wish to have your food delivered or have an office-mate pick it up for you when he or she goes out to eat. Pick someone who eats regularly and in a healthy manner.

Who do I know who fits this job? _____,

_____, and _____ .

8. You can get home cooking if you make a trade with someone who will do the cooking for you. In exchange you might babysit, do carpentry repair, or do yard work for the person.

Here's a list of five people who I can contact to make a trade. And here's what I can trade:

Person   Trade

_____   _____

_____   _____

_____   _____

_____   _____

_____   _____

9. If you don't mind cooking but don't want to mess with cooking every day, make enough to feed yourself and your family for a week. Maybe you cook two chickens or several pounds of meat, make a batch of rice and a batch of potatoes. You can even make a huge salad, omitting the dressing, and store it.

What do you choose to make the first week? _____

_____

Store each type of food separately and freeze part of it in individual containers. Have side dishes or condiments that change the flavor: barbeque, ethnic variations, or whatever you like.

When you're preparing to leave for the day (or night), place some of the frozen food in a container that you can place in a microwave or oven. You may wish to put a topping on at that time.

When you're ready to eat, heat it or pull it out of the refrigerator, add dressing or condiments, and you have your meal.

For practice, I will try this for two weeks. _____yes

10. Keep healthy food snacks on hand at work and at home such as nuts, seeds, dried or fresh fruit, or cheese.
I prefer these snacks: _____
_____

11. As for sleep, you would do well to look closely at your own natural rhythm.
When do you prefer to sleep? _____night _____day
Do you like to take short naps? _____yes _____no
Though there are programs that attempt to retrain people to fit the standard eight-to-five daytime schedule, you will end up using a lot of time and energy trying to change yourself from who you are, especially over time. It will tend to stress your system.

12. You may wish a drastic change in your schedule to fit your body's rhythms. Consider night work, if you're a night person.
I would like to change my schedule to _____ .

13. If you feel that it is okay to be the way you are, but you need to adapt to a schedule for a while that doesn't fit, how can you change the time you go to bed or get up? For example, if you have classes that meet in the early morning, but you're a night person, could you go right home after class and go to sleep, and then do your homework after you wake up, staying awake until after class?
The plan I'd like to try out is _____
_____ .

14. You must disregard people who say you *should* sleep a particular number of hours a night or at a certain time. Healthy people's sleep habits vary greatly. Let's say you only need a few hours of sleep a night. Someone voices a different opinion of what you should do. You can tell the person, "Thank you for your concern, but I'm in charge of my sleeping."
I am willing to face someone politely and tell them I know what I am doing. _____yes

Your Commitments:

I commit to seek my natural rhythms.	_____yes
I commit to variation in my food.	_____yes
I commit to be kind to my body, giving it plenty of quality rest.	_____yes

What Makes This Hard To Do:

Believing that there is a *right* time and way to sleep and eat presses you into a pattern that is *wrong* for you. You must counteract this belief by standing up for what the True You naturally responds to. Discover the means that fit you.

2

Following Through to Success

Practical, everyday life teaches us to keep our eye on our goal, if we are to succeed. Yet do we not often feel we've failed to achieve our goals in a timely manner, getting off track or not traveling in the straight line that we've been taught is the way to achieve outcomes?

Brainstyle not only shapes the nature of the goals that interest us but the manner in which we strive toward them. For some of us, the shortest, fastest straight-line approach may work well. But for many others of us, providing a broader range of experience as we travel to the goal not only better fits our innate brainstyle but yields the kind of end product we desire.

This section urges the True You to become sensitive to alternative ways to achieve the goals you desire. Guidelines to avoid getting and staying off track because of the particular way in which you do things will help the Accommodating You avoid stress and loss. Best of all, new hope for successful follow-through to goals you previously thought were out of reach will allow you to enjoy the success of accomplishment.

MAKING A BIG PURCHASE

Question:

Do you feel you're *supposed* to do research before making a big purchase?

Why This Happens:

- Not everyone has the same natural approach to making a big purchase. Your way may not be to do "research" first.
- You have an approach to life that is shaped primarily by your feelings. You experience the styles and tones of things. You are likely to relate to the patterns created by what you see and the relationships between what you see and what is around them. Your partner may approach life in a 180-degree opposite way. Thus when you approach a purchase with that person, you may have different ways of making the selection.
- You may feel embarrassed or guilty because the culture in which you live teaches that practical details are more important than feelings and aesthetics.

Problems You Face Making a Big Purchase:

- You may go right out and begin to look at items in which you are interested while your partner may turn to research Internet sites to try to find out which is the best, most efficient, or valued selection you might make.
- Right away you begin to disagree about how the other is going about the selection.
- Even if you're making your selection alone, others tell you that you *should* research the item and you feel inadequate and embarrassed when you don't want to do this.
- You get confused and feel desperate because you fear you shouldn't trust your feelings.
- You end up getting something that you don't really like, though it may be practical. That hurts your heart.

Your Goal:

To work as a team with a partner who approaches such situations differently than you do, act sensibly, and get what you want and like.

What Not To Do:

Do not feel bad or superior about the way in which you go about making a decision.

Your Work:

1. When making a big purchase, it is important to make use of the brainstyles of the people involved in the decision. The range of the brainstyles may vary from extremely linear to extremely analog, yet you want to work together with a balanced approach.
   I want to work toward achieving a balanced approach. _____yes

2. If you're working with someone with a brainstyle different from yours, you must take the other person's brainstyle into account without giving up on the way your brainstyle works.
   I agree to take another person's style into account while simultaneously honoring my style. _____yes _____no

3. If you answer "no," why won't you? Are you afraid an argument or power struggle will develop?
   I do fear problems such as an argument or power struggle. _____yes
   I do not want to work with the other person because _____
   _____ .

4. If there are problems in your relationship, you need to learn to negotiate before you try to make a joint decision. Preferably ask the other person to join you in the learning.
   I am willing to learn to negotiate. _____yes
   When I asked my partner to also learn negotiation skill he/she said _____
   _____ .

   If your partner doesn't want to join you, consider learning yourself, but be prepared for the possibility that you will have little ability to make a big purchase jointly without considerable strife.

5. Choose a purchase you want to make jointly. Investigate the market in a way that is comfortable for you. Each of you may have different ways of gaining information about what you want to purchase. You may want to shop around looking for what attracts you. Your partner may want to check *Consumer Reports*, the Internet, and systematically gather information.

I like to approach a big purchase by _____
_____ .
My partner likes to approach a big purchase by _____
_____ .
Remember, neither way is right or wrong. You simply approach making selections and purchases differently.

6. Sit down with your partner to negotiate the important issues about the purchase regardless of how you got your information. Share what each of you considers is important when considering the purchase. You will need to take turns leading the discussion. When your partner leads, he or she needs to take charge of listing all the particulars that need to be considered from the vantage point that comes easily for him or her.
I am willing for my partner to list his or her wishes first.
_____yes

7. As you read or listen to the other person's list, you will learn what is important to that person.
I am willing to learn what is important to my partner.
_____yes
Here is what is on my partner's list: _____
_____ .
Now make your own list and then let your partner read it.
Here is the list of what's important to me: _____
_____ .

8. Draw out each other's preferences. Note what you each feel adamant about and what you can do without.
My partner feels strongly about _____ .
I feel strongly about _____ .
My partner can do without _____ .
I can do without _____ .

9. It is extremely important that neither of you puts down the other's suggestions or wishes.
I agree to not put down my partner's wishes or suggestions.
_____yes

10. Do not let anyone put your needs down, even when they're based on feelings. You can see that this does not happen by simply saying "My needs are important to me, and I will see that I go about getting them met in my own way."
I will not let anyone put my needs down. _____yes
I can say the following to anyone who tries: _____
_____ .

11. If your partner continually judges your wishes and ways of doing things, you probably are dealing with someone who has control issues. You will then either need to give in or seek counseling to get beyond the control problems that undoubtedly plague other areas of your relationship.
I choose to give in. _____ yes
I choose to seek relationship counseling. _____ yes

12. Say to your partner, "I want you to get your needs met, too. We'll find a way even if it takes a while."
I commit to seek a consensus about our purchase. _____ yes
I expect my partner to do the same. _____ yes

13. If you're making a selection alone but hear others' messages in your head, simply say to yourself, "I'll take responsibility for the way I do things. I appreciate the input, but my final choice will have to please me." Now write this down:

_____
_____
_____ .

14. Realize that any decision is not a forever decision. Everyone learns over time to be practical. When you make an error, you are not bad, irresponsible, or incompetent. You will learn.
I am willing to learn from past experience regarding the selection of any big purchase. _____ yes

Your Commitments:

I commit to letting my heart lead me in my selections.   _____ yes
I will also factor in practical issues.   _____ yes
I will commit to take another's viewpoints into account
  and find a way to honor my feelings and needs and the
  other person's at the same time.   _____ yes

What Makes This Hard To Do:

Decision making can become very emotional, especially when two people have markedly different styles of brain construction. Even people who love each other often may have distinctly different preferences. It will take mutual caring, understanding, and creativity to bridge the gap that opens between the way you each go about making big decisions.

FAILING TO FOLLOW THROUGH

Question:

Do you feel that you fail to follow through on chores?

Why This Happens:

- The most common reason for lack of follow-through is that you have committed to do something you *should* do but don't want to do.
- You may be a person who has a lot of interest in relationships—more interest in talking to people than in spending the time doing what you've talked about doing.
- You may live in the here and now, especially on your days off, flowing through your day, one moment at a time, with your focus on the present rather than on some future goal. As a result, you lose contact with your goal.

Problems You Face Because You Fail to Follow Through:

- You make plans that you don't follow through on.
- You don't get your chores and "have to's" done.
- You let other people down incurring disappointment or anger.

Your Goal:

To get done what you commit to and only commit to what you're willing to do.

What Not To Do:

You don't want to set yourself up to feel guilty, and you don't want to let others down.

Your Work:

1. In order to successfully follow through, you must only commit to doing something that you are truly willing to do.
   I will watch carefully that I only commit to doing things I am truly willing to do. _____yes
2. You must be honest and strong with other people, especially family and friends, so that you say "no" if someone asks you to do something you don't want to do.

I want to be strong and fully honest about what I am willing to do. _____yes

3. Empathetic, sensitive people often agree to do things to please people even when they don't want to do them.
   I will be very careful not to agree to do things even when I want someone's approval or feel their disappointment at being turned down. _____yes

4. You can empathize with someone you turn down about being able to help problem-solve their needs as a substitute for doing the job yourself. You may say, "I wish I could help you, but I just don't have the time or resources. But let's think of alternative ways for you to get what you need."
   I can do and say this. _____yes

5. When you are bullied or otherwise threatened into saying you will do something you don't want to do, you are being set up to not follow through. You can say, "Pressuring me won't help. I could tell you I will do what you want just to get you off my back, but I won't follow through. I could, however, help you come up with an alternative."
   I will watch out for this kind of pressure and set my own limits. _____yes

6. Assess yourself and your wishes before you agree to do something. Ask yourself questions such as the following:
   How do I want to use my time on my day off? _____
   _____
   How do I feel about doing chores? _____
   _____

7. Sometimes you just want to "go with the flow" as a way to relax. When you feel this way, should you commit to doing a task at a specific time?
   I will not commit to do a specific task at a specific time if I want to relax. _____yes

8. If you tell someone you will do a chore and you later realize you don't want to do it, you need to go the person and explain how you feel. Apologize and then say what you will do.
   When I change my mind, I will let the person know and explain how I feel. _____yes

9. If the person you're thinking about is likely to give you a hard time over your change of heart or change of time, you need to be prepared to address the resistance. If you usually follow

through, just say, "I'm sorry I committed to you this time. I'll be more careful in the future."

10. Ask yourself if you change your mind frequently. If you do, you need to stop it. Sure, you may do it out of fear or a desire to please, but those are not valid excuses. You must commit to stop letting yourself and others down.
Yes, I often change my mind, which has the effect of letting the person down. I will work hard on changing this habit. _____yes

11. If you habitually fail to follow through, you may need to be responsible by following through even though it is a hardship on you. This will help teach you to not commit to things you may not later want to do.
I agree to take responsibility to follow through on things I commit to do so that I break the habit of saying I'll do something and then changing my mind. _____yes

12. Remember, you also can participate in finding alternative ways to help that person get what he or she wants, such as hiring the job out or making a trade with someone you know.
Some things I have to trade, including money, to get jobs done, are _____

_____

13. If the chore is urgent, see if you can make the chore or task bearable to do. For example, you may find that creating a "work crew" of friends who help one another in emergencies combines camaraderie with doing the job. Think of an urgent/important chore that really needs to get done and that you don't want to do and design a "crew effort."

_____

_____ .

14. If you have the financial resources, you may need to give yourself permission to hire someone to do the chore for you.
I am willing to hire someone to do the job I don't want to do. _____yes _____no

Your Commitments:

I commit to follow through on tasks I commit to doing.   _____yes
I commit to continue to take responsibility to see that
   tasks are accomplished even if I don't do them myself. _____yes

I commit to only accept those tasks that I am willing
   to do or for which I will take responsibility.   _____yes

What Makes This Hard To Do:

The cultural ethic that puts work before play or relaxation may leave you feeling guilty. You are neither *bad* nor irresponsible because you choose to do something you want to do. Simply express your own value system and understand that not everyone will like it. You need not go along with what others believe is right, but be kind and thoughtful as you negotiate the practical matters of life.

LIMITING YOUR LOSSES

Question:

Do you regularly burn pots, lose contact lenses, or overflow the backyard pond because you don't pay attention to what you're doing?

Why This Happens:

- Any task that has a beginning and an end with nothing for you to do but wait in between means trouble. If you are an active person, doing nothing while you wait is next to impossible.
- If you do a task at intervals rather than repetitively, you will find it hard to develop a pattern that keeps attention focused during the waiting period.
- Cleaning a contact lens is a job that requires you to use only two fingers to rub the cleaning solution on the lens for a few seconds. Your eyes, ears, and other hand are free to do *something* during those seconds. It only takes a second or two, after all, to move things around in the medicine cabinet. Or you start to wash the sink or put the cap back on the toothpaste. It's during the times of extra activity that you drop the lens or it flies out of your hand, never to be seen again.

Problems You Face Because of Your Losses From Your Lack of Attention:

- You waste money, materials, and time because of your lack of attention to what you're doing.
- Others get angry with you because of your wastefulness.
- You endanger your home or property.
- You feel guilty because of your irresponsibility.

Your Goal:

You want to become less wasteful, take better care of your things and the people in your life, and don't want to be a threat to the environment or those in your life. You want to get control of your attention while you're waiting for something to finish.

What Not To Do:

Do not beat up on yourself or think you are irresponsible because your attention flags while you're waiting for something to finish getting done.

Your Work:

1. If the True You is a lively, creative person who enjoys doing many things, you may not be fully able to solve this problem. Look for a solution that will reduce the frequency of your losses.

   Though I may not fully solve my attention problems, I want to find ways to reduce the frequency of my losses. _____yes _____no

   I accept that, because of my brainstyle, I may not be able to be as good at keeping my attention focused while I'm waiting for something to finish as people with a different brainstyle. _____yes _____no

   If you answer "no," consider the reason for your answer. Consider the following possible explanations.

   Do I judge my behavior as being bad or wrong? _____yes

   Have I been told that there is something *wrong* with me because I forget to turn off things? _____yes

   Who has said these things about me? _____

2. What habit do you want to work on first?

   I will work on _____.

   I accept that it may take a week or more to work on changing this habit. _____yes

3. You must discover something that will call your attention back onto the task during the period you are waiting. For example, in the case of a teakettle on the stove, you may get a kettle that whistles loudly, so the whistle is your cue to *do something immediately, NOW!*

   I will immediately act when _____ happens. _____yes

   Remember, if you ignore the cue, even for a second or two, you run the risk of forgetting it alerted you. Gentle timer beeps are far too easy to ignore and forget.

4. With a short task like cleaning your contact lenses, where you only have seconds to wait, you must commit to do nothing

that is active. Here are some ideas of what you can do instead. Add more of your own.

I can:

stare at my fingers	_____yes
count numbers in my mind	_____yes
sing a short tune	_____yes
repeat a phrase	_____yes
_____	_____yes
_____	_____yes

Know that you are instilling a money-saving habit. Give yourself a treat for your work after the behavior is habituated.

I will treat myself to _____ .

These new habits probably won't last indefinitely. You will require a refresher course periodically to reinforce something that is not natural for your style of brain construction. But the reminder won't take as long to reinstall as it did in the beginning.

I will schedule the repeater course (date) _____ .

I will write it on my calendar. _____yes

Your Commitments:

I commit to do the best I can to change habits that cost
me money, time, or effort.   _____yes
I also commit to change so I do not put other people out. _____yes
I commit to be both self-accepting and responsible at the
same time.   _____yes

What Makes This Hard To Do:

Establishing a habit that is not natural for you is difficult. Be patient with yourself. Solutions are not permanent, so remember to reinforce the habit regularly.

TUNING OUT

Question:

Do you say "Uh-huh" and fail to follow through on your commitment?

Why This Happens:

- Some people do a lot of thinking. Conversations run through their heads and they watch movie-like scenarios in their minds.
- If the True You is a big-picture person who becomes wholly absorbed in what you're doing or thinking so that you become one with it, you may not perceive something said to you in a regular voice. This happens especially if you're busy, have a lot on your mind, or are watching TV.
- Specifically, what happens is that when you're addressed, you have a high enough level of attention to respond automatically with "Uh-huh," but not high enough to translate your response into action. You do not follow through because you didn't get the communication strongly enough to turn your agreement into action.

Problems You Face Because You Tune Out:

- Others get irritable or angry with you because they think you've committed to something that you haven't even fully heard.
- Others think you're irresponsible about following through on commitments.
- You are unaware of your behavior and so are helpless to fix it.

Your Goal:

You need to be clear to those with whom you communicate about what it means when you say "Uh-huh" and ask for their help so the relationship runs smoothly.

What Not To Do:

Do not continue to let other people down because of your level of attention.

Your Work:

1. Enlist the assistance of each person with whom you have a relationship, business or personal. Consider people to whom you say "Uh-huh" in your personal and work life.
    I will ask the following people to help me with my attention:

    _____   _____
    _____   _____
    _____   _____

2. Tell each person that you may say "Uh-huh" to a request without mentally registering the request strongly enough to do it.
    I agree to tell each person to whom I say "Uh-huh" without following through that I may not actually register his or her request enough to do what they ask, though I would be willing to do it. _____yes
    Place a check by the names of the above people as you tell them.

3. Also say, "I'd very much like to do whatever you ask," assuming you do. "I'd like to know when I tune out, but don't know I've done it. Will you help me?"
    I agree to speak further to each person. _____yes
    Place a second check by the names of the people you've talked further with.

4. Directly ask each person if he or she is willing to work with you. If someone, usually an angry spouse, says he or she is tired of your dependency and refuses to work with you, know that there is more wrong with the relationship than this one issue. Fill in the person's name and circle agreement or unwillingness to work with you.

    _____ is/is not willing to work with me.
    _____ is/is not willing to work with me.
    _____ is/is not willing to work with me.

5. Do not accept criticism or scolding from a person and don't expect that person to be able to be on your team.
    At this time I will not try to convince someone who has lost trust in me to help me when I say "Uh-huh." _____yes

6. Suggest a willing helper (secretary, spouse, or friend) stop you when he or she needs something from you. Tell the person to touch you, call your name, or nicely ask you to repeat the request by saying, "What did I just tell you?" Or ask them to

get your attention with questions like *"When* will you bring me the file?" or *"When* will you take out the trash?"
I prefer my helper to:
_____touch me _____call my name _____repeat their request

7. If you're asked, "What did I say?" immediately after you said, "Uh-huh," you'll probably be able to answer. But let a second or two pass and you won't be able to recall the request.

8. Check to be sure that you don't say "Uh-huh" as a diversionary tactic to get someone off your back.
I agree to not use "Uh-huh" when I don't want to do something. _____yes

9. Be sure to say "thank you" to those willing to help you.
I will be sure to say "thank you" to those willing to help me. _____yes

Your Commitments:

I commit to take responsibility for my lack of
attention. _____yes
I am willing to do all I can to improve the situation. _____yes
I commit to let others know how grateful I am for
their help. _____yes

What Makes This Hard To Do:

If you or someone else feels you are being irresponsible and blames or shames you for your lack of awareness, you are likely to get into arguments. Bad feelings and emotional sparring will likely take the place of genuine problem-solving and teamwork. Don't engage in this nonconstructive behavior.

ANCHORING A DRIFTING MIND

Question:

Does your mind ever drift from what you are reading or from listening to someone who is speaking to you?

Why This Happens:

- As a person whose brain focuses on the interconnections and relationships between things more than on specific bits of information, you are likely to drift away from one thought to a complex of thoughts. That's just how you're made. You quickly and automatically connect what you hear with what you already know and start to think about it.
- Something we read, see, hear, or otherwise perceive draws our attention to think about or feel about it as it applies to us. This happens when you are a kinesthetic learner. You become very involved in what you are doing and *begin to live* the experience. So, if you are reading about geology, you may begin to think about how much you like turquoise and how you'd like to go to Arizona to learn to do silversmithing so you can make jewelry.
- You may also begin to have feelings that pull you off track. For example, your boss is telling you about your next assignment, and you begin to feel scared that you won't be able to accomplish it. You become all tied up in your feelings of fear and your mind stops listening to what your boss is saying.
- You may become bored, already knowing what the writer or speaker is going to say. Taking too long to get to the point annoys you. Worse yet, your mind drifts as you think about other things, waiting for the sentence to end.
- You become distracted by your own body's needs or by something you see or hear in the environment.

Problems You Face Because of a Drifting Mind:

- You are reading and the next thing you know you're at the bottom of the page and don't have a clue what you just read.
- You are listening to someone speak, but then can't answer a question he or she asks you because your mind has drifted.

- You tune out when someone goes into too much detail or talks too slowly.
- You fail to take in what teachers and trainers are saying because you stop listening at some point.
- You fail to hear directions or requests that are important.

Your Goal:

To learn to anchor your attention so you won't stay "off track" and miss critical information.

What Not To Do:

Please don't beat up on yourself or feel helpless because your mind drifts.

Your Work:

1. In order to affect the problem, you must begin to tell yourself that you can develop the skill of noticing when your mind drifts.

   I can develop the skills I need. _____yes

2. Let's say you are reading. As soon as you become aware of your mind drifting, place your finger on the place in the book where you begin to think about something other than what you are reading.

   As soon as I am aware of my mind drifting, I will place my finger on the place in the book where I stopped paying attention. _____yes

3. Next, jot down a note or draw a picture in the column of the book or on a nearby notepaper of what you were thinking. This will remind you of your intervening thought. Start reading a page right now and practice this technique.

   In the column of the book, I will make a note as soon as I realize my mind has drifted. _____yes

4. To anchor this skill, you must commit to return to your note later. In this way you honor your creative thinking by paying attention to your notes.

   I commit to return to the note later. _____yes

   What does the note say? Write it here. Or draw the picture you made.

_____
_____
_____
_____
_____ .

5. If your mind drifts during a conversation, ask the person to repeat what was just said. There's nothing wrong with this. If you ask with confidence, it's usually perceived as a compliment. It's even okay to mention that your mind drifted. You might say, "I started thinking about what you were talking about and need you to repeat the last thing you said. I don't want to miss anything you said."
   I agree to practice this as soon as I can. _____yes

6. As a person speaks to you, you can anchor your mind by repeating to yourself what the person is saying. Or every couple of sentences you can repeat a part of phrase back to the speaker that he or she has just said. That will keep you attentive to the conversation.
   I will practice these skills. _____yes
   Later, I will summarize the effectiveness of these suggestions.

_____
_____
_____ .

7. If you begin to feel an emotion that is distracting you, note the feeling instantly and commit to return your attention to it later when you can analyze it without interrupting your attention to the speaker.
   I am willing to become aware of what I am feeling and to analyze my feelings later. _____yes

8. Physical reinforcement will help you pay attention. You can nod your head slightly to a speaker, affirming to yourself that you are paying attention. Look the speaker in the eye.
   I will express my attention physically during conversations. _____yes

9. As a member of an audience, ask for clarification as soon as you fail to understand something because of your drifting attention. You may say, "Excuse me for interrupting. I want to be sure I understand what you are saying." This is a compliment.
   I will be able to practice this technique at the following meeting: _____
   _____to be held (date) _____ .

10. If you're becoming bored, grit your teeth, play a rhythmic tune with your toes on the inside of your shoes, or do anything that is quiet and not disruptive.

The best thing for me to do to pay attention even when I'm bored is _____.

11. If your body's needs are distracting you because you're hungry or tired of sitting, or you notice some other discomfort, pat yourself and reassure yourself that you'll attend to the need as soon as possible. Even better, prepare ahead of time. You know that you need to take something to discreetly nibble on, have a drink handy if possible, or sit so that you can stand up and move around at the back or side of the room if your body gets tense from sitting.

I can carry _____ with me to hold me over and I will make sure that I am able to stretch or move about without distracting the speaker. _____yes

12. If you're distracted by an outside interference, you may wish to request a change that will reduce the distraction for everyone. Perhaps the window or door can be closed. You can even suggest a change of room.

I am willing to take a leadership role in a group if I notice a disruptive influence that is distracting me or the group. I know I won't be the only one who is bothered. _____yes

13. If you're not engaged in a dialogue but are a listener, having something in your hands can stimulate your alertness. This could be a paper clip, handiwork, or a pencil and paper on which to doodle or take notes.

I prefer to take _____ with me to help me focus my attention on the speaker.

Your Commitments:

I commit to learn the skills to anchor my mind while reading and listening.   _____yes

I commit to take a leadership role in seeing that I get the best possible outcome to situations requiring my attention.   _____yes

What Makes This Hard To Do:

It takes practice to get through to your attention in order to learn new habits. You must tell yourself you can do it. *And you must practice for a while.* Whenever possible, avoid truly boring situations.

RETURNING TO COLLEGE

Question:

Are you worried that you'll never be able to get the higher education you need to do what you want to do in life?

Why This Happens:

- As a sensitive, big-picture, kinesthetic learning person who takes in everything at once, entering any new educational level can be overwhelming. That may be what happened if you went to college right after high school—going from a structured environment to one that is chaotic and requires self-structuring while demanding a high level of performance. Also for the first time you may have had to take in all the requirements for living, socializing, and being on your own in addition to mastering your course work. That's enough to overwhelm anyone with a brainstyle like yours.
- There were likely too many options to face regarding what to study and the kinds of interests to pursue. Confusion was probably the result.
- College programs teach students using only a fraction of the types of intelligence available for learning. They tend to favor linear learners who can memorize facts and take tests well. So, you may not have worked up to your intellectual potential.
- The first time a kinesthetic, sensitive, big-picture person tackles a large new enterprise, the results often are less than wonderful. But after you've run through the routine, you will have a much clearer idea of what to expect and how to handle the situation. As a result, you're likely to do much better the second time around.

Problems You Face As a Returning Student:

- You may have had a failure the first time you attempted higher education, so you're worried you'll fail again.
- You are unable to get the kind of job you would like and be good at because it requires higher education.
- Book work may have always been really difficult because you're a kinesthetic learner.
- You feel overwhelmed by all the new things you have to attend to by returning to school.

Your Goal:

To follow your dreams by successfully continuing your education.

What Not To Do:

Do not panic that you'll have a repeat performance of an earlier failure.

Your Work:

1. Begin by noting the difference in yourself since you first attempted college.
   I am different now than I was when I went to college before.
   _____yes
   Before I was _____
   _____.
   Now I am _____
   _____.

2. You may find it is helpful to start a journal or have a conversation with another person about your college voyage. Find a mentor, if you can, who believes in you.
   I would prefer to _____journal, _____have a conversation, _____do both.
   I would like _____ to be my mentor. I will ask him/her (date) _____.

3. Write and talk about your current reasons and goals for going to college.
   The reason I am going back to college is _____
   _____.
   My goals for college are _____
   _____.

4. Look for colleges and training programs that are nontraditional, inventive, and offer "credit for experience" programs. You may find guides in the resource section of your public library and in high school counseling offices as well as the Internet. Community colleges often serve as excellent re-entry institutions to begin higher education.
   Resources that I plan to use include: _____
   _____
   _____
   _____.

5. Talk with a New Student Counselor or a counselor for students with special needs. Special needs categories include Attention Deficit Disorder as well as returning students. You probably qualify on both counts.
   I will speak with the following people:
   Name _____ Location and phone _____
   _____ _____
   _____ _____
   _____ _____
   _____ _____

6. You may wish to consider utilizing the Americans with Disabilities Act. Remember that having an ADD brainstyle doesn't mean you're disabled. It means that your style of learning may not fit the academic style of teaching. You need an equal opportunity to learn what you're capable of learning and the opportunity to prove you know what you know. That's where the Americans with Disabilities Act comes in. (See "The Americans with Disabilities Act" at the end of this book.)
   I plan to check out the Americans with Disabilities Act.
   _____yes

7. When you return to school, you will be wise to take small classes and a light load at first.
   I plan to take _____ number of college hours my first semester/quarter. I can increase this as I feel comfortable.
   _____yes

8. Do not worry about grades. Instead, focus on getting the degree, the power credential, you want and get on out of school as soon as you are able.
   I like the idea of getting out of school so I can apply what I've learned. Application is my strong suit. _____yes

9. Stay focused on one semester or quarter at a time. Though you will occasionally need or want to look at the big picture, that can be overwhelming, so don't do it very often. Take college one step at a time. This is particularly important for returning students who often have their own families and frequently have to earn a living while attending college.
   Besides going to school, I have other things in my life. They are: _____
   _____
   _____ .
   I agree to take college one step at a time. _____yes

10. Select your professors carefully. Be sure to choose those who teach using communication methods that you understand.
    I agree to choose professors carefully. _____yes

11. If you get into a class in which you can't understand what's going on, withdraw immediately and search for a professor with a different teaching style.
    Be sure to withdraw immediately so you don't end up with a failing grade.
    I commit to withdraw immediately. _____yes
    I feel _____ about withdrawing from a class.

12. You may be tempted to feel like you are the one who is a failure because you couldn't understand or get along with the professor. That's fine to consider, but don't jump to that conclusion. It might just as well be the presentation style of the professor. At any rate, there's no need to find fault or blame anyone. There's just a mis-fitting learning/teaching situation.
    It's hard for me to not blame myself.   _____yes
    I am willing to consider that maybe I am
        in a situation that doesn't fit my
        learning style.   _____yes
    I'll talk to a counselor, fellow students, and
        other teachers to try to analyze my
        difficulties.   _____yes

13. Get to know your professors and teachers in your areas of interest. Often, they can help you from behind the scenes to get through classes that are difficult for you.
    I will spend time getting acquainted with my professors and teachers and will ask for help as needed. _____yes

14. Seriously consider using tutors and study groups for subjects that are difficult for you.
    I will use tutors and study groups as needed. _____yes

15. Consider finding ways to work in the job area that interests you while you are in school. This will reinforce your interests in classroom work and motivate you to stay in school. You are also likely to find mentors in job settings who will encourage and help you.
    Jobs that will help me maintain my interest and motivation might be _____
    _____
    _____.

16. Though your main focus is on getting an education, don't forget to have some fun and take R & R along the way or you will become susceptible to burnout. Follow your sense of whether you want to take a semester off. It depends upon whether you think you can get back on track afterwards.
Fun and R & R I would enjoy while in school are _____.
I believe I _____could _____could not take a semester off while going to school without hurting myself.

Your Commitments:

I commit to do the best I can to reenter the
academic environment.   _____yes
I commit to keeping a balanced approach to my
studies, do what I can, and let go of what
doesn't fit me.   _____yes
I commit to find the help I need to succeed.   _____yes

What Makes This Hard To Do:

Because much college work for a kinesthetic learner is like trying to run a marathon with a fifty-pound weight on each leg, you may become discouraged. If you do, take a little time off. Also consider other avenues that will allow you to do what you love. There is often more than one route to your goal. You may need to change majors rather than give up your dream.

3

Behaving Yourself

The style of your brain construction often dictates the kinds of behaviors you struggle to overcome. In this chapter you'll learn that there is not one right way to be or do things in order to get what you want. You'll find ways that can work for you because they follow the nature of the True You.

Temper, impulsivity, and getting a "high" are all behaviors that make foreheads crease with a scowl. These and many other behaviors fall outside the limits of acceptable social conduct. Yet these are forms of communication that are carrying a message of need. For example, instead of using words to express "I'm afraid. I need to feel protected," a temper outburst surrounds a person with a layer of protection, creating an illusion of safety.

But the price of unacceptable behavior is high and the efficiency of meeting the actual inner need is low. When the True You is naturally active—verbally, mentally, and physically—you are also likely to find that your behavior spills over the boundaries of *acceptable* behavior.

What a relief to become aware of some of the many opportunities you have to gain not only clarity into why you behave as you do but also options to get your needs met without incurring a high price tag. Learning to stay true to yourself while remaining within the parameters established by social limits allows you to win along all fronts in the best interest of yourself and those around you.

You'll learn to live in a world that requires self-responsibility, communication, and thoughtfulness of others even when it also demands that you accommodate it in ways that don't readily fit you. Spending time living according to the values in which you believe will stop further personal wounding as well as the wounding of others as you take charge of your behavior. The Accommodating You can and will discover how to bridge the difference.

The True You, working with the Accommodating You, will find ways to hold down your end of a task while finding ways to support the way your brain is constructed. You'll be able to let others know what you need and what you can give. Everyone ends up a winner.

HANDLING CHANGE

Question:

Do you dislike change, mostly because you fall apart when you are confronted with it?

Why This Happens:

- As a big-picture, kinesthetic person who takes in everything around you *all at once*, you suffer enormous overload when you are confronted with changes. Everything is new.
- When the True You lives by patterns—that is, the relationships between things more than details—change brings problems. Change creates a breakup of the old patterns that guided you. In addition, it takes you a while to see the new patterns because they are made of a lot of details. To establish new habits and integrate them into new patterns takes time. So you are left initially with no way to structure what you are experiencing.
- As someone who doesn't organize according to details, often not knowing what to initially do with individual occurrences, you are suddenly attacked by a myriad of new things.
- If you're sensitive, you will *feel* your discomfort intensely.
- To the degree to which you take things personally, you may think that what is happening to you is personal. You may feel as if you are the only one who gets so upset, reacts so poorly, or feels so badly.
- All change causes all people to have to adjust.
- When change happens *to* you, it's usually more unsettling than if you create it.
- The effects of change are cumulative. If you've had a lot of change recently, you are likely to have failed to recover from early stresses before incurring new ones. Pretty soon you're awash in stress.

Problems You Face When You Change:

- You have difficulties adapting to a new job, lifestyle, or activity.
- You become overwhelmed by too much to do too quickly.
- You grieve the loss of old friends and old ways.

- Your energy declines, leaving you less effective at accomplishing all the new requirements.
- Your eating and sleeping habits suffer.
- You may become irritable or depressed.
- You start thinking negatively about the new way and your ability to pull off what you are facing.

Your Goal:

To learn to handle the results of change so you learn from them rather than get wounded by them.

What Not To Do:

Do not rush into your new situation and ignore your need to let your body, mind, and emotions adjust at their own rate.

Your Work:

1. At first, simplify your life by only doing exactly what you *have* to do.
   Knowing I have to simplify, here are the things I *have* to attend to: _____
   _____ .

2. Get extra hours of sleep. Be sure you eat healthy food regularly. Take refreshing breaks (naps) even when it means you don't get things done.
   Normally I need _____ hours of sleep a night, but now, with all the change in my life, I feel I need _____ hours a night. I _____do _____don't like to nap. I will let myself take _____ number of naps a day.
   I also will make sure I eat more nutritious but easy-to-obtain food. This is no time to try new recipes. _____yes

3. Slow down. Do not rush. Do not take on new tasks or try to be creative until you've stabilized your life. So that you won't feel that you'll *never* get around to what brings you joy in life, make a list of things you'll get to when you have regained your equilibrium.
   When I am used to the changes in my life so they no longer feel new, I will return to doing _____ .
   And I will also begin to _____
   _____ .

4. Make lists, getting all the details out of your head of the new things you must accomplish as well as the old ways that you need to resurrect. But don't think you have to accomplish the whole list at once. Be cautious not to become overwhelmed because as a big-picture person, you see everything you have to do to fill in the big picture the way you want it to become.
Things I want to do over the first month: _____
_____.
Things I want to do over the first three months: _____
_____.
Things I want to do over the first year: _____
_____.
Now double the amount of time you are planning to spend accomplishing these goals.

5. Most people rush, thinking they must get everything organized in the first month or so. It takes a minimum of six months to a year or two to rebalance in relation to big life changes. If you've also undergone a loss (such as a divorce or death), it will take closer to two to three years. List the losses or changes that affected your transition.
Changes and losses that occurred in my life that are a part of my needing to make changes in my lifestyle are _____
_____.

6. Set priorities. Maybe time with your family comes first. Learning your new job comes next. Time for yourself is lower on the priority list for now. Add in time to work on your new home. Hanging pictures may be way down on the list along with other nonessentials unless you feel adrift without them. Go back to the list of things you jotted down that you want to do over the next months and put a number after each item in order of importance to you.

7. If, for whatever reason, your change does not turn out to be satisfactory after you've given yourself time to adjust, don't stay stuck just because of concern for what others might think. Even if you initiated the change, move on. There's little way of knowing how things will work out until you live with the choices you make. Resist the adage "You made your bed, now lie in it." Remember, kinesthetic learners learn by doing, that is, by trying out situations. Only then can you tell how something will work for you and how you will feel about it.

I agree to give myself permission to evaluate
my changes after a period of adjustment.   _____yes
I can change again, if I need to for my peace
of mind and prosperity.   _____yes
I will resist others' opinions about my decisions.
I will do what is in my own best interest.   _____yes

Your Commitments:

I commit to slowing down and treating myself
carefully as I adjust to the changes in my life.   _____yes
I will feel pride in simply surviving the changes
in my life.   _____yes
I will give myself permission to change my mind
as needed.   _____yes

What Makes This Hard To Do:

Most people rush through change, failing to realize how strenuous
it is. Family and friends may insert their opinions regarding your
adjustment period. Tell them "Thank you," then do what your
mind, body, and emotions are telling you is the right thing to do for
you at a given time.

TAKING CONTROL OF YOUR IMPULSIVITY

Question:

Do you do things without thinking?

Why This Happens:

- Driven by feelings more than thoughts, you may try to please someone or take care of something by quickly doing whatever you feel will help.
- If you have a long-standing habit of shortchanging yourself by focusing on others exclusively, forgetting what you need, you will likely act impulsively and suffer as a result. Suffering wounds you.
- Your sensitivity to another's needs may drive you to do something before you've had time to think through a plan of action and implement it.
- To the degree to which the True You is a kinesthetic person and a doer, you'll tend to find your solutions by acting them out. You really don't learn by being told what to do but, instead, you do learn from experience, unless you're shamed, which increases anxiety and sets you up to act even more impulsively. Left unassaulted by shame, you probably will be more careful next time you're in a situation that caused you trouble before.
- Impulsivity tends to be present when you feel you cannot get what you need. As a result, when you see even a tiny opening on the pathway to get what you need, you jump at it.
- If your impulsivity leads to clumsiness, it's not so much that you're innately clumsy. It's more that you're quickly trying to do two or more things at once. For example, you're reacting to your feelings *and* taking action at the same time.

Problems You Face Because of Your Impulsivity:

- Your impulsivity creates accidents.
- You hurt others and yourself without meaning to.
- You feel foolish or even ashamed because of the impulsive things you do.

Your Goal:

To curb your impulsivity while still getting your needs met.

What Not To Do:

Do not continue to let your impulsive tendencies express themselves unchecked.

Your Work:

1. You can get your needs met while honoring the True You. If the Wounded You feels fearful in this respect, say to yourself, "I'll learn to get my needs met without hurting myself." Write this as a reminder to yourself and carry it in your purse or billfold.

   _____

2. Envision yourself as someone who has a natural rhythm—one that can smoothly and skillfully guide you through your daily activities.
   I visualize myself in this way. _____yes

3. Recall how you were raised, and refashion your beliefs about yourself to achieve a new, positive self-image. See yourself as you want to be.
   I visualize myself as I want to be. It looks like _____
   _____ .

4. Affirm to yourself that you can learn to get your actions under your control.
   I can get my actions under control. _____yes

5. Now, practice taking a breath before you act. Breathe easily and steadily.
   Say, "I breathe—in and out, in and out." (Write this) _____
   _____
   Say, "I take a breath before I act." (Write this)_____
   _____

6. Look for specific triggers that cue you to act. One common trigger is trying to please someone else. Another trigger is feeling ashamed or inadequate. By analyzing past impulsive acts, you will begin to be more aware of the emotional or situational triggers that get you in trouble. List three times in the past when you acted impulsively and then recall and write down what you were feeling just prior to the act.

Impulsive Act 1: I was _____
_____ .

Impulsive Act 1: I felt _____
_____ .

Impulsive Act 2: I was _____
_____ .

Impulsive Act 2: I felt _____
_____ .

Impulsive Act 3: I was _____
_____ .

Impulsive Act 3: I felt _____
_____ .

7. To deal with a trigger such as wanting to please another person, tell yourself that it's okay to want to please someone else, but not at your expense.
I will please another when I want to, but not at my expense. _____yes

8. Congratulate yourself for even the smallest improvement. Taking one step at a time will get you where you want to go.
I congratulate myself. _____yes

Your Commitments:

I commit to look at myself in a different, improved way, ignoring what others have said about me over the years.   _____yes

I commit to tell others who still criticize me that I am gaining control over my behavior and would appreciate their support. But if they can't give it, I would ask them to say nothing.   _____yes

What Makes This Hard To Do:

Lack of awareness of the emotional and situational triggers that precede impulsive acts makes it hard to change impulsive behavior. Habits, long ago formed, take time to change.

SHIFTING GEARS AND BEING INTERRUPTED

Question:

Does it drive you crazy to have to change from one task to another or be interrupted when you are involved in a task?

Why This Happens:

- The attention regulator in your brain tends to have two settings, on and off. Often there's no in-between, so it's difficult to readily shift from one thing to another either because you're interrupted or because the task requires you to change direction.
- You also are likely to see the big picture, the completed project you're working on. You may see the "best possible scenario" for whatever you are doing. You want to get to these projections before you quit working.
- You may be able to do only one thing at a time. It could even be hard for you to deal with more than one relationship at a time.

Problems You Face Because Shifting Gears and Being Interrupted are Hard for You To Do:

- You may feel quite emotional when you have to shift gears or are interrupted.
- You may be hard for others to be around.
- You probably find it hard to get back on track after the interruption.
- Your efficiency level goes down when you have to shift from one task to another.
- Losing sleep and not refueling your body with food as needed are side effects that compromise your health and well-being.

Your Goal:

To be able to more smoothly shift gears and not feel so upset because of it.

What Not To Do:

Don't blow up or blow a task off because you have trouble shifting gears when you are interrupted or need to change direction.

Your Work:

1. Engage in self-study. You may also want to ask a parent or sibling for input.
    I will also ask _____ to help me. _____yes
    Here are some questions for you to use to assess yourself.

    Am I aware of my reactions to being interrupted
        or changing tasks?   _____yes
    Do I feel stressed under these conditions?   _____yes
    Has it always been hard for me even in childhood?   _____yes
    Have I tended to do one thing at a time?   _____yes
    Have I tended to have one relationship at a time?   _____yes
    Do I do better concentrating on only one subject
        or task until it is completed than juggling
        several at a time?   _____yes

2. Because transition times are often very difficult for you, you need to be particularly aware of any demands coming from outside your current focus.

    Think of a current project that you're engaged in. What demands—personal and professional—surround you that you usually have to pay attention to, that irritate you, or that cause you to have problems?
    I can think of several things that usually cause me trouble:
    _____
    _____
    _____ .

3. Interpersonal relations are often affected when you have trouble changing from one thing to another. When your needs are different from those of others, explain how you work.
    I will speak with those people in my life who are affected by my trouble changing gears. _____yes
    They include (name them): _____, _____,
    _____, _____, _____ .

4. Set specific limits on yourself, allowing extra time to change from one task to another. For example, if you are organizing your kitchen during the day wearing sloppy clothes, and then plan to go out to dinner in the evening, you'll need to allow extra time to stop your daytime activity. You'll need extra time for the transition required to clean up and change clothes. It's up to you to take responsibility to stop *on time* rather than expecting another person to have to wait on you.

I am willing to take the responsibility to both stop what I'm doing so that I have the time for a transition and factor in enough time to make the transition. _____yes

I will allow _____ time to change from one activity to another.

5. Once you've committed to a reasonable schedule, make plans for how to mark the place where you stopped. This could, for example, be a red bow on the kitchen cabinet you just worked on. It might be a list with completed items crossed off using a colored pen. Or you might lay your pen across the line where you want to return to work. Think of a project that you may need to interrupt.

That project is _____

_____ .

First, I would like to try _____ to mark the project when I need to stop working on it because of an interruption.

6. Reassure yourself that you'll complete your task by setting the time when you'll return to it.

I will return to my project _____.

7. You may decide at times to ask others to not interrupt you during a project that is important to you. Explain to anyone you're involved with about your need to stay with the task. Tell the person how you'll help them to remember. Say, "I'll put up a sign that says, 'No interruptions, please.'" Or say gently, "Not now. I'll be taking a break at _____." Or, "Can we talk tomorrow?"

Ask them to not disturb your uncompleted project. Thank them in advance and again later for helping you so they understand how important it is to you.

I will tell the people around me that I am going to put up a sign asking them to not interrupt me until I'm finished with my task. And I will thank them in advance. _____yes

8. If you are in a situation such as a timed exam that requires you to quickly shift from one section to another, you may need to ask for accommodation to take the sections separately allowing time for transition from one to another. (See the Addendum: The Americans with Disabilities Act, at the back of this book.)

I will become familiar with the accommodations available through ADA and will use them as needed. _____yes

Your Commitments:

I commit to do the best I can to take responsibility for the way in which my brain is structured that causes me to have trouble shifting gears and objecting to being disrupted.	_____yes
I commit to ask others to help me.	_____yes
I also commit to be more tolerant of disruptions even though they bother me.	_____yes

What Makes This Hard To Do:

You are likely to suffer greatly or even find it impossible to follow anyone else's time frame because it's so hard for you to get back on task after being interrupted. As a result you may have developed habits, such as blowing up, that take time to re-educate. But you can do it.

HAVING A TEMPER OUTBURST

Question:

Are you known for having a temper?

Why This Happens:

- Anyone can have a temper outburst when he or she is under enough stress. A temper display is protective covering for feelings of helplessness and vulnerability. It may happen when you don't get something you badly want or are hurt or startled.
- People who are sensitive are vulnerable and more likely to get hurt, so they often throw up a temper shield for protection.
- Temper expressions can become habits. When your temper outburst has provided you with what you wanted, having a temper outburst easily becomes a habit. Even when you've been repeatedly scolded for blowing up, your temper was reinforced and became habituated. The problem is that the price of having a temper is high even when you get a payoff, as tempers are exhausting. Also, other people may get tired of being around your temper displays and scold you. They may even begin to reject you.
- Kinesthetic people act out their anger tangibly in observable ways such as slamming doors, yelling, cursing, and driving too fast. If you are a kinesthetic person, you run a high likelihood of having an observable temper.
- If you fear you will not get your basic needs met, you may cover your fear with a temper outburst.

Problems You Face Because of Your Temper:

- You hurt or alienate the people you love.
- You are denied good service and outcomes, hurting yourself.
- Your reputation suffers, personally and on the job.
- You lose business and jobs because of your temper.
- You may get in trouble with the law.

Your Goal:

To get your temper under your control so it doesn't rule you.

What Not To Do:

Do not continue to allow yourself to let your temper control you.

Your Work:

1. Because a temper often erupts to protect you from threats, you must find alternative ways to protect yourself that don't cost so much. Make a pledge to yourself that you'll find new ways to self-protect and get your needs met.
I pledge that I will work to find alternative way to protect myself. _____yes

2. Think about the last time your temper got out of control.
I can recall the last time my temper got out of control. It looked like this:

_____

_____.

3. Ask yourself what happened immediately before your outburst. That event served as a trigger for your temper. You will be able to use this awareness to head off further temper outbursts.
Right before my temper erupted, _____

_____

_____.

I understand that what I've described served as a trigger for my temper. _____yes
Everyone has specific "hot buttons." When these are touched, even lightly, you are more vulnerable to react strongly. For example, if you have an especially strong need to please others, you'll be more susceptible to situations that get in the way of your gaining that approval. Think of the last time you attempted to please someone. Describe the situation and what happened afterwards.
The last time I tried to please _____, the following happened: _____

_____.

4. Sometimes you may be fearful that someone won't accept you unless you please him or her. If you feel this way, you are in a position to lose a lot of emotional security. This is a set up for a temper outburst.
I feel fearful I won't be able to please someone important to me.
_____yes
The last time I tried, my temper _____.

5. To curb your temper, make a purposeful decision to work on it. This means finding ways to attend to the inner needs that lie behind your temper.

   I agree to work on my temper. _____yes

6. Become watchful of situations that trigger your temper. Especially notice when you're feeling stressed, in a hurry, or fearful of an outcome.

   I get stressed when I am in a hurry and may
   lose my temper.   _____yes

   I have lost my temper when I'm fearful of
   an outcome.   _____yes

   It happened when _____
   _____.

7. You may have lost your temper when you were hungry or lonely or tired.

   I am susceptible of losing my temper when I'm:
   _____ hungry _____ lonely _____ tired

8. The key to mastering your temper is bringing your hidden needs out in the open. Tell someone you can confide in about them. You may need to do some counseling work at this point. Know it takes courage to face your inner vulnerabilities. The reward is worth it.

   Here's what I need to feel okay: _____
   _____.

   If I need to, I commit to meet with a counselor to help me learn what I need and what to do about what I need.

                                                       _____yes

9. You may also make a list of other ways to protect yourself besides blowing up.

   I can think of different ways to self-protect and feel empowered besides blowing up. Here are some of them: _____
   _____
   _____.

10. If someone feeds your temper by giving in to you or nagging and scolding you when you blow up, tell that person you are working to change and ask them to refrain. They may or may not be able to respect your request.

    I have someone in my life who feeds my temper by nagging and scolding me until I blow up. _____yes

    That person is _____.

This is what happened the last time I blew up at the person:

_____

_____.

I will ask that person to stop nagging and scolding. _____yes

11. Only you can be responsible for stopping your temper behavior. But if you're being reinforced by someone, you may have to decide to back away from that person if he/she can't stop reinforcing your nonconstructive habit.

When I asked the person to stop nagging or scolding or giving in to me, he/she did/said _____

_____.

Now that I know the problem with the person, I can get control of my temper and still be around that person.

_____yes

I will have to back away from the person.   _____yes

12. Congratulate yourself when you make headway. Though expecting perfection right away is not realistic, watch for little gains and be proud of yourself.

I congratulate myself because of the headway
   I've made.   _____yes

I'm proud of what I've done so far.   _____yes

Your Commitments:

I commit to work on my temper.   _____yes

I am surrounding myself with people who can help
   me more than hinder me in achieving my goal.   _____yes

I commit to learn many ways to get my needs met
   other than by using my temper.   _____yes

What Makes This Hard To Do:

The hardest part of getting a temper under control is dealing with someone who sabotages your progress by being involved with your temper demands. You may also find tough going if you believe you can't get your needs met except by having a temper outburst.

DISPLACING YOUR ANGER ONTO OTHERS

Question:

Do you displace your anger onto people you love?

Why This Happens:

- If you are in a situation where you can get in trouble because you are angry at a person, especially an authority, you (like most of us) are likely to bottle up your temper. Parents, bosses, teachers, and police are examples of such authorities.
- But the anger doesn't go away because you've kept it inside. If anything, it actually becomes stronger.
- When you come around someone whom you do not fear, such as a loved one, or with someone whom you have no connection, the anger is likely to come out. Kicking the dog, fighting with someone weaker than you, or snapping at a stranger such as a clerk are examples of this. Road rage reflects displacement of anger. You know it when someone shoots the finger at you for a driving infraction or cuts in and out of traffic, coming dangerously close to creating accidents with other drivers even when there is no driving-related cause. These are extremely dangerous situations and the best advice is to get as far away from the angry person as you can.

Problems You Face Because of Displaced Anger:

- You may threaten your safety or that of others.
- You can jeopardize your personal relationships by inappropriately placing blame on those who are emotionally safe.
- Displaced anger doesn't really truly relieve you of the anger or its causes. It can actually add more stress to you and your health.
- You can alienate those who are willing to be "on your team," who play a supportive role in your life.

Your Goal:

To get back in charge of your life and your emotions.

What Not To Do:

Do not displace your anger on others, spreading your temper.

Your Work:

1. Begin to get in control of your temper by recognizing what you're doing and commit to stop displacing your anger onto other people and situations.
   I humbly accept that I have a problem with my temper.

   _____yes

   I am not *bad* because of it.   _____yes
   But I do have to stop displacing it onto others.   _____yes
   I commit to stop displacing it onto others.   _____yes

2. Pay attention to the causes of your anger. That's what will help you get control of yourself.
   Look at the last three times you became angry and list what caused the anger.
   The last three times I became angry, I _____
   _____
   _____ .

3. When you assess the causes of your anger, do not blame it on someone else. No one is *making* you angry. A person may do something you don't like and you feel angry. But the anger is a cover-up emotion that arises to keep you from feeling helpless, frightened, hopeless, or frustrated. You must uncover the true emotion under the angry feelings. Identify the underlying emotion in each event you describe.
   When I consider the last three times I became angry, underneath the anger was a feeling of being 1. _____,
   2. _____, and 3. _____ .

4. Next, consider whether you can work out the situations that are causing you to become angry. Ask yourself if you think you can rectify the situations if you talk in a professional or calm manner to the person involved. Knowing about the problem, the person may be able to change, and you'll feel better. Many times people don't know that they made someone angry.
   Situation 1. I believe I might be able to rectify the situation if I talk to _____. _____yes _____no
   Situation 2. I believe I might be able to rectify the situation if I talk to _____. _____yes _____no
   Situation 3. I believe I might be able to rectify the situation if I talk to _____. _____yes _____no

5. If you answered "no," believing that the person may not be able to change, know it was worth a try to consider asking.

I am willing to try to talk to someone who makes me angry even though it will only work some of the time. _____yes

6. When you do approach a person whom you feel anger toward, do so calmly with a plan for how to change the situation. Always have a plan to suggest rather than going to the person to complain.

Here's a plan I've developed for what I might say for each of the three situations with which I'm working.

Situation 1. _____

_____ .

Situation 2. _____

_____ .

Situation 3. _____

_____ .

7. If you are in a situation that is destructive, you can expect to feel angry. Assess the cost of staying in it if no changes are possible. Caution must be used whether you decide to stay or leave it.

I am currently in a situation that is destructive to me. It looks like this: _____

_____ .

8. Consider if you are staying because you're afraid of change. Do you see yourself as inadequate?

What is the cost of my staying? _____

_____

If you are afraid or feel inadequate, you have a place to begin to work so that you can live up to your True Self with its potential. Consider what you have to offer.

Though I feel inadequate, I see that I have several things to offer wherever I go. They are: _____

_____ .

If you leave, you may lose income for a time; others may not understand or may disagree with you.

What is the cost of my leaving? _____

_____

9. Having considered the costs involved, you can now decide whether to leave now or later or stay indefinitely. What do you choose? Do not be in a great rush to decide, but do decide one way or the other in a reasonable amount of time so you can get on with your life.

I choose to _____stay, _____leave right away, _____leave by _____ (date).

10. Until you either resolve the issue or are able to leave the hurtful situation, consider ways to turn your angry energy into something constructive, either at work or outside, instead of displacing it where it doesn't belong.

You may become competitive, generating additional business on the job.

You might channel your emotions into inventive and creative challenges as you focus on problems that have gone unsolved. You may express your anger artistically.

Consider physically working off your angry energy by running, engaging in athletics, chopping wood, digging in the garden, or pursuing strenuous activity.

I will channel my anger in the following ways instead of displacing it where it doesn't belong: _____

_____

_____.

11. Make sure that you don't bottle your anger up inside of yourself, turning it into depression. That is not a healthy way to handle it. It indicates that you will have to do something about your situation. Signs of depression include feeling down, worthless, or helpless with lowered self-esteem. Your eating and sleeping may change. Your health may begin to deteriorate. Your total energy may be diminished.

I have the following signs of depression: _____

_____

_____.

I will change my situation myself and/or seek counseling for my depression. _____yes

But know that medication to alleviate the depression without changing the cause of the internalized anger is not a long-term solution. You must change your situation.

Your Commitments:

I commit to cease blaming others when I feel
angry and will seek the true feeling underneath
the anger I feel.   _____yes

I will cease displacing anger on others that needs to
be worked out in relation to someone else.   _____yes

I commit to taking action that is in my best interest.   _____yes

I will be responsible for taking the action without
hurting others, even those with whom I'm angry.   _____yes

What Makes This Hard To Do:

To get back in charge of your life, you'll need to resolve old emotional issues that caused you pain in the past and will cause you to face that pain now. You'll also have to change long-standing habits. These are hard jobs, but not unbearable ones, and the results are well worth the effort on your part.

LIVING WITH UNEXPRESSED ANGER

Question:

Do you feel at a loss about what to do when you can't safely express your angry feelings?

Why This Happens:

- Being confined in a situation means you have no tangible power, no matter how powerful you were at earlier times or how emotionally powerful you may still be. This leads to a high level of stress.
- Being trapped in a situation that you simply can't give yourself permission to leave, such as caring for a chronically ill family member, places enormous pressure on a caregiver. It creates feelings of helplessness.
- Since feeling helpless or vulnerable is one of the underlying reasons for a temper to be triggered, your fear of a temper outburst is well taken. And if you will either get in trouble or feel terrible if you discharge the temper, you are faced with the need to find alternative ways to survive.

Problems You Face Because You Can't Express Feelings of Anger:

- You may be punished for expressing your temper.
- You may feel terribly guilty if you express your temper.
- You may compromise your physical health.
- You may become significantly depressed.

Your Goal:

To learn to do something with your temper when you can't safely express it.

What Not To Do:

Do not think your situation is hopeless. Do not hurt yourself.

Your Work:

1. Facing the underlying causes for your reactions is the one thing you can do in a situation when you can't express your

anger. You must look deeply within yourself to the source of your fear, helplessness, hopelessness, and frustration. You are looking at the feelings that feed your temper. You must do this tenaciously, but gently.

I will gently look at the feelings underneath my angry emotions. _____yes

2. You may want to try writing your feelings down. Or you may find talking them out with another person or in a group is more to your liking. You may also wish to seek counseling to explore the feelings and memories that underlie your temper. Either or all of these options will be a big help.

I will write my feelings down.   _____yes
I will talk about my feelings:
   with another person   _____yes
   or in a group.   _____yes
I will seek counseling to help me work
   through my feelings.   _____yes

3. If it was unsafe for you to express your angry feelings as a child, you would have learned to inhibit their expression. Recall when you had an angry feeling as a child. Visualize the child part of you in your mind or recall the scene.

As a child I recall a time when I felt angry but didn't feel safe expressing my feelings. This was the situation: _____
_____ .

4. Ask what it was that you needed at the time.

I needed _____
_____ .

5. Do not chide yourself for wanting or needing something then, even if all your memories are of people telling you that you shouldn't need it.

If I find that I scolded myself in my vision or in the past, I'll stand up to that scolding part and tell it to stop. I and my child part don't deserve it and don't need it. I will be my own advocate. _____yes

6. Now begin to think of ways to help your child part express his or her feelings. What did you want to say?

I wanted to say _____
_____ .
He/she needed _____ .

7. Next rewrite the early scenario in your mind or in a journal, seeing your grown-up self helping your child part get what you needed. If that was impossible, visualize your child expressing appropriate anger. Make the story you write supportive and fulfilling for the child.
The rewrite of my past looks like this: _____
_____
_____ .

8. Continue to raise that child part of yourself, showing options so that your child part has more than one way to get his or her needs met, even currently in a difficult situation. Be very self-nurturing. Commit to staying with the child part of you.
I realize that rewriting my past experience isn't the end of the job I have to do to continue to keep my temper under control. I will be self-nurturing as I need it. _____yes

9. Project your new imagery technique for expressing your feelings and getting your needs met into some future scenario so that you'll have some practice in constructively facing future situations when they occur. Mentally practice conquering the kinds of situations that used to cause you trouble. Even as you're confronted with a currently stressful situation that taxes you, acknowledge inwardly to the child part of you that you understand the stress and will stay with your child part. Tell yourself that you are sending support.

You will notice you experience a lightening of the pressure within you. It doesn't fix or even change the external situation, but it does change the effect on you, giving you relief and perspective. You'll feel better.
I can visualize a future scenario where I'm likely to see no way to change the limitations on my life. But now I have a way to support the child part of me, my feelings-part. I give myself permission to express my feelings and I acknowledge the needs and wishes I have. _____yes

Your Commitments:

I commit to take care of my inner emotional needs
by being understanding and self-supporting.   _____yes
I commit to work with my own feelings rather than
lose my temper at someone else.   _____yes

What Makes This Hard To Do:

The hardest part of changing the habit of a hot temper is not believing you'll be able to learn constructive ways to get what you want and need. Because you learned helplessness in this regard from a very young age, it will take time and practice to learn new habits. But you can do it!

RESPONDING TO DISRESPECT

Question:

Does it make you so angry when someone treats you or a loved one with disrespect that you go on the offensive?

Why This Happens:

- As a sensitive person who feels everything keenly, you will tend to feel deeply about anything in which you place value. This includes the belief that people ought to treat each other with respect.
- Being ordered to do something instead of being asked is overkill when you are a person who is loyal, sensitive, and has a good track record. It feels insulting and tends to create a need to throw up a defensive shield to cover hurt. When you're simply asked to do something, it's amazing how cooperative you and people like you become.
- If you tend to be a feeling person, you lead with your feelings, feeling first and thinking later. Even though some of your buddies may be able to brush hurtful, demeaning things off, you will take it personally and *feel* terrible about it. (See "Taking Things Personally" in chapter 4.)
- To the degree to which you are a people-pleaser, you will try to do the best you can for anyone you admire. But if you don't admire another's behavior, you either get depressed or want to retaliate.
- If you are self-monitoring, someone judging or evaluating you or another person feels awful, and you want to fight back.

Problems You Face Because You're Sensitive to Disrespect:

- You hate it when someone scolds or criticizes you or someone else. It tears you up emotionally.
- You get angry and yell or stomp around when you are disrespected.
- You hurt all over when someone disrespects you or someone else.
- You argue even when you don't have power in a situation.

Your Goal:

To be less affected by disrespectful behavior, scolding, and criticism and be able to curb your reaction to it.

What Not To Do:

Do not overreact or openly respond to a troublesome situation until you have had time to think how you want to handle it.

Your Work:

1. It's in your best interest to learn to look at situations with perspective as if you are watching what is happening from a distance.
   I realize I need to get some emotional distance
       from situations that are hurtful.   _____yes
   I am willing to work on doing this.   _____yes

2. Clearly distinguish between your personal feelings and the event. This requires you to use your thinking mind in conjunction with your feelings. Think of the last time you felt someone was disrespectful, critical, or scolding to you.
   I recall the time and can describe what happened: _____
   _____
   _____ .
   I recall thinking _____
   _____ .
   And I felt _____
   _____ .

3. Looking back at the example you chose, engage your thinking mind and review what happened to kick off your feelings. This will establish the link between your feelings and your thinking—an important link.
   I see the link between my feelings and my thinking. It looks like _____
   _____ .

4. Next, turn your attention to the person you see as being disrespectful. Analyze what might be happening to the other person. For example, maybe he is zealous about his job, fearful he will not do it well enough. Maybe he's always been treated harshly and doesn't know any other way to be with people. Or maybe she's never been treated with respect. Maybe her job power has gone to her head.

Reconsidering the person who was disrespectful to me, I *think* he/she might have been/is _____

_____

_____ .

5. Find ways to self-protect that won't get you in trouble, such as whispering your irritation to a trusted companion. You might also make jokes about the situation after you leave. The stand-up comic in you may have found great resource material. More on the serious side, you might compose a memo or e-mail either to your boss or the other person's boss. Tell about the incident and ask for help in resolving it. Add that you believe both of you are valuable to the company and you'd like to improve relations. Include any suggestions you think of for a better way to handle the situation.

I can imagine trying _____

_____

_____ .

6. Know what kind of power you have. No matter how wonderful your value system or how honest, forthright, or cooperative you are, others can't tell that until they get to know you. If they have more tangible power than you, you'll need to concede to them, at least until they can get to know you. Anyone, even an emotionally powerless person who has more job-related power than you, will have power *over* you. You need to factor this in when you're deciding what to do.

Does the person I'm thinking of have tangible power
over me?   _____yes
Does that person have high emotional power?   _____yes
Do I have more emotional power than the person? _____yes

7. If you're dealing with someone who has authority over you or someone who is not interpersonally insightful, you may choose to say nothing. But assess what the person can handle and then decide if you want to work directly with the person on the issue. Never try to get through to someone who doesn't have the skill to know what you're talking about.

I believe that the person I'm concerned with _____ does _____ does not have the ability to be insightful about the situation.

8. To defend yourself against the pain of being ordered about, criticized, or scolded, check to see whether you asked for the input or not. Be cautious not to ask someone for help or ask for an opinion unless you're willing to take whatever he or she gives you. A lot of people think that a request means you *want* criticism. Let the person know clearly what you want from him or her.

   I know someone who thinks any request means a request for criticism. This person's name is _____ and my relationship with the person is _____ .
   I will make a point to not ask for that person's opinion unless I want criticism. _____yes

9. By the way, it's okay to ask for someone to tell you your work is wonderful. You can even say that. "Just tell me my work is wonderful." This is a good thing to do if you've had a bad day or feel beaten up. A variation is: "I don't want criticism. I just want you to tell me what this piece says to you."

   If someone is demanding, scolding, or critical, you can simply say, "I don't appreciate what you're saying." Then back away. You have control over unwanted criticism.
   I can use these approaches to solicit input for my productions and creations. _____yes

10. If the person with whom you are in contact regularly continues to use a scolding tone with you, know that some people sound that way because of their past experience. They may not even know they sound that way. You can feel sorry for the person, which will help you feel better. You can ask, "Are you intending to scold me?" If the person says "no," continue, "I feel as if you are." You might want to add, "I don't do well when I'm scolded or criticized. I'd appreciate your changing your tone."
    I can do this. _____yes _____no _____ I'd prefer not to say anything.

11. Own up to any errors you've made, saying, "Though I may have made a mistake or didn't do something the way you would have liked me to do it, I'm not willing to be scolded for the job I've done. You can tell me what you want. I'll do my best." Your own tone needs to be moderate and free of scolding to pull this off.

I can imagine saying this to someone who
    bothers me.   _____yes
I will ask someone I trust to tell me the truth
    about whether my tone of voice is scolding.   _____yes
The person I'll ask is _____ .

Your Commitments:

I will treat other people with respect.   _____yes
I commit to avoid criticizing and scolding others.   _____yes
I will not let another scold or criticize me. I will
    handle the situation calmly and firmly.   _____yes

What Makes This Hard To Do:

You must overcome the tendency to react immediately to a disrespectful situation. That takes training so you'll need to practice.

Many people truly believe you *should* not be so sensitive and
ought to get past your sensitivity. But consider whether you want
to dull the beautiful sensitivity you have and can use in your behalf
in other kinds of situations. Instead, develop new ways to deal with
disrespectful and harsh situations.

FINDING WAYS TO SIT STILL

Question:

Do you find it hard to sit still?

Why This Happens:

- Your physical activity level is naturally high.
- You're naturally expressive and probably a kinesthetic learner, so you learn and work better when you are moving a part or all of your body.
- Required to sit for long periods of time, you are likely to feel physical pain. You move to relieve the discomfort.

Problems You Face Sitting Still:

- Though you are not moving in response to anyone else, another person may feel the effect of your moving and may take it personally. You aren't *doing* it *to* the other but that person may feel bad because of your activity level.
- Western culture seems to believe that "stillness is better than activity" in many situations, such as learning and office environments. In other settings, high activity levels are acceptable and even desired.

Your Goal:

You will want to work with situations that cause you trouble without attempting to become a quiet person.

What Not To Do:

Don't let your high activity level control you and draw attention to you if you don't want it to.

Your Work:

1. You need to learn ways to accommodate your activity level so you are comfortable and do not bother others.
   I will learn this for myself and for the benefit of others.

   _____yes
2. You must accept your need for movement. (Hummingbirds don't apologize for being very active.)

Upon thinking rationally about my need for movement, I realize there is nothing wrong with me. I accept my need.
_____yes

3. You need to prepare yourself ahead of time to avert problems caused by your activity level.
I now remind myself that I must think ahead about situations that I am going to face, analyzing them with regard to the constraints on my movement. I will do this. _____yes
I will look for situations where activity is acceptable.
_____yes

4. Your planning is two-fold. You must also figure ways to move that won't bother others.
I also do not want to bother others, so will seek ways around this while getting my needs met. _____yes

5. Look for situations that easily can be adapted to your activity level or even that will benefit from it. Here are some examples. Check them off if they may be beneficial for you.
   • Get an outside job that allows you to move around all day. Examples include a job in outside sales or gardening, as a courier, or athlete.
   • Whether you're in your office or at the movies, choose chairs/stools that swivel and rock.
   • Sit near the back of rooms so you can unobtrusively get up, walk around, or lean against a wall or doorjamb.

6. Keep something with you to "fiddle with." Be sure it doesn't make noise. Examples:
   • A paper clip or rubber band you can twist in your pocket.
   • Plastic beads suspended between two knots on a leather thong.
   • A wand with viscous liquid and particles to rotate.
   • Handiwork—Feel free to tell the speaker that you listen better if you are doing something with your hands.
   • Draw a picture.

7. Do an activity that is quiet but serves the purpose of letting you move.
   • Take notes even if you never look at them afterwards.
   • Learn a silent resistance exercise technique such as isometrics.
   • If you swing your crossed foot up and down, cross your ankles and wiggle your toes inside your shoes.
   • Play music with your toes or fingertips.

- Use trips to the drinking fountain or restroom when you need a movement break.
- Above all, don't work longer than your "sitting span" will comfortably allow.
- Other suggestions: _____
_____.

I will try the following: _____
_____.

Your Commitments:

I commit to follow through with this plan.   _____yes
I will begin to work my plan (insert date).   _____
I will continue to work on this plan in the following way: _____
_____
_____.

What Makes This Hard To Do:

One of the hardest parts of keeping still is believing that any motion is wrong. Small unobtrusive motions that relieve your stress and do not bother those around you are the answer.

QUIETING A NOISY MIND

Question:

Do you have a mind that chatters, thinks, and is constantly imagining all sorts of things?

Why This Happens:

- As a sensitive person, you will notice and absorb large amounts of stimulation from your environment. Subjected to so much input, you will find your mind filling to capacity. Your sensitivity also extends to noticing what you feel emotionally and physically from your own body.
- If you have experienced trauma or difficult emotional experiences, you will likely have a large amount of posttraumatic images, sounds, and feelings as your mind tries to make sense of them and heal you.
- Without a way to drain off, organize, or release this input, it will tend to chaotically churn about in your mind.
- When you are excited by or even focused on a project, you will tend to stir up even more creative ideas as you see the many implications of each strand of your thinking. This happens when the True You has a predominantly analog style of brain construction that automatically networks and connects lots of details into patterns.

Problems You Face Because of Your Noisy Mind:

- You are distracted by the images and thinking that goes on in your mind so that you are inefficient at work.
- You have trouble sleeping because it's hard to turn your mind off.
- You get tired because of everything that is booming and buzzing around in your mind.
- You get confused by the different mental activities you experience.

Your Goal:

To quiet your mind by first using natural means to direct, utilize, and calm the flow in your mind.

What Not To Do:

Neither allow this mental busy-ness to wear you out nor medicate it into stillness without working first with natural means to direct, utilize, and calm the flow.

Your Work:

1. Begin by gently searching for quieter, less stimulating environments in which to place yourself and find natural, healthy ways to soothe and calm your mind.

   You can begin to work on your environment first or you can begin to discover ways to calm your mind. Or you can do both simultaneously.
   I would like to begin to
   _____work on my environment
   _____find ways to calm my mind
   _____both

2. When you begin to work with your environment, assess the amount of stimulation in your environment. Spend a day or two noticing your surroundings. Pay attention to sounds, movements, reflections, colors, and textures. Utilize all your senses—sight, hearing, smell, taste, and touch.
   I will notice with my senses:
   Hearing—sounds and noises_____

   _____
   Sight—patterns, items, people, and movement _____

   _____
   Smell—smells _____

   _____
   Touch—textures and pressures _____

   _____
   Taste—how things affect me that I eat or ingest _____

   _____

3. There are also your gut-level feelings that pick up the emotional tone of your environment. You may feel them physically in your body or through your emotions. You may be surprised to discover you are exposing yourself to a variety of feeling tones—tense, frenetic, angry, soothing, joyful, fearful, or a multitude of other emotional tones. Remember, your sensitivity is one of your strongest suits. It can work for you or against you. Be aware.

Gut-level feelings that I become aware of: _____
_____ .

4. Analyze and evaluate each type of stimulus you receive. Consider asking yourself a series of questions about each.
   Is the sound around me noisy or soft sounding? _____
   Is it pleasant or irritating? _____
   Is there a lot of movement in my environment that I can see, hear, or feel? What is it? _____
   _____ .
   Is it predictable or unpredictable? _____ .
   Do I find the movement pleasant or unpleasant? _____
   Are the patterns I see busy, blended, rigid, geometrical, or other? _____
   _____
   Do I like or dislike the patterns that surround me? _____
   Are there many or a few colors surrounding me? _____
   Do the colors harmonize, clash, soothe, or agitate? _____
   Am I surrounded by one of my favorite colors in a hue I like?
   _____yes
   Am I surrounded by any colors I dislike? _____yes
   What are the textures to which I'm exposed? _____
   Can I physically feel them? _____yes
   Do the textures feel pleasant or unpleasant? _____
   Is the environment natural or manufactured? _____
   Do I prefer one over the other, and how do I feel in the one I like the best and the one I like the least? _____
   _____
   Do I prefer to be inside or outside? _____
   Do I spend more time inside or outside? _____
   Do I prefer a rural or an urban environment? _____
   Which do I work in? _____ Which do I live in? _____
5. Note how many aspects of your environment please you.
6. If many displease you, what can you do about them? Ask yourself how much control you have over your surroundings. Be specific.
   How much control do I have over my surroundings? _____
   _____
7. If you are lacking in control, what little things can you do to improve your comfort? And is this enough?
   I can change _____ .
   Is this enough? _____yes _____no

If you answer "no," visualize a setting in your mind that is pleasing. Visualize it any time your mind needs quieting.
The setting that will help calm my mind looks like _____
_____ .

8. If you have some or a lot of control over your environment, how can you make it more agreeable for you? Consider ways in which you can calm down your environment or smooth it out so your mind is less stimulated. Many people are put on mental overload by working in the city. They find country living a necessity and a pleasure. Certain sounds bring calm to people. Some folks like the ongoing sound of the sea while others like the steady drum of traffic and city life. Find your own preferences and work to spend as much time as possible in the ones you like.
My ideal environment in which to spend work time looks and feels like this: _____
_____ .
My ideal environment in which to relax or play looks like this: _____ .

9. Another way to quiet down your mind is to consider using a CD player or tape recorder with earplugs through which you can listen to the sounds you like.
I would like to use a _____ and listen to _____
_____ .

10. Still another way to calm your mind is to try meditation. It is an excellent way to acquire mental calmness. This does not necessarily mean an "empty your mind" form of meditation. For active minds, this is not a realistic goal. Guided meditation often works well with busy-minded people. There are CDs, audio tapes, and training programs available to assist you in finding what works best for you. Sample them until you find what works for you.
Here are some of the meditation experiences I plan to try:
_____
_____ .

11. Yoga is also a good way to combine breathing with motion in a calming way. Before long, you will find that you are actually doing a form of meditation while you're doing the yoga routines.
I would like to try yoga to help me learn to quiet my mind.
_____yes

12. Certain tones and sounds are soothing. In particular you may be drawn to the sounds of nature, such as live birds (especially cooing doves), running water, wind in trees, frogs croaking, and so on. On the other hand, you might feel calmed by totally different sounds. Rock and roll works for some people.
I would like to try _____
_____ .

13. Mental visualization of pleasant scenes helps many folks meditate. If you have fond memories from childhood, pull these up into your mind's eye. Or create a fantasy scene or replicate one you've noticed in the movies or on TV.
The next time my mind starts buzzing, I'll do a mental visualization. _____yes
One scene I'd like to visualize is _____
_____ .

14. Massage, polarity, and cranial sacral therapy as well as other forms of bodywork utilized on a regular basis can do wonders to relax your mind.
I would like to try a form of bodywork to quiet my mind. _____yes

15. Activities such as gardening, long-distance running, fishing, and working on a potter's wheel calm some people. Try being out of doors close to the earth or water to feel the calming of nature. There are many activities from which to choose. What they generally have in common is some repetitive motion or their ability to sooth.
I like _____ to quiet my mind.

16. Journaling or drawing pictures of your thoughts may also effectively remove them from your mind.
I like the idea of journaling.   _____yes
I already journal.   _____yes
I like the idea of drawing or painting what's
   in my mind.   _____yes
I already use artwork as a tool in my life.   _____yes

Your Commitments:

I honor the activity in my mind and know I can guide the
   activity from confusion to usefulness.   _____yes

I commit to find ways to quiet my mind so I can
    use the content in my own best interest.   _____yes
I will try a wide variety of things to gain that
    control, knowing that my uniqueness spreads
    to finding the way that fits me as I am.   _____yes

What Makes This Hard To Do:

It can take time to make environmental changes. And it takes time
to work with your own inner processes to find what's soothing for
you. Sometimes major life changes are necessary if you are to find
a fit for the True You, but the results can be extremely satisfying.
Life is too short to continually expose yourself to environments
that don't fit.

Taking the time to train your own inner mind is worth every
moment you put into it. It's ranked up there with good nutrition
and physical fitness.

Caution:

If you suffer from obsessive thinking in which the *same* thoughts
repeat over and over and over in your mind, you would do well to
consult a professional who treats this type of disturbance to your
well-being.

TALKING LOTS AND LOTS

Question:

Do you talk incessantly?

Why This Happens:

- Just like some people are typically very physically active, some people are verbally active.
- The amount of talking anyone does also depends on the environment in which he or she's been raised. So if you were raised in a family whose members talk a lot, you are likely to feel comfortable talking—unless, of course, no one ever listened to you.
- If you were not taught to listen as well as talk, you may not realize that you over-talk or "hog the stage," leaving no room for dialogue.
- Different situations determine the amount of talking that is useful. A friendly off-hours conversation can go on for hours while on-the-job, bottom-line interchanges need to be succinct. A problem will arise if you don't distinguish between settings.
- Sometimes people talk endlessly in an attempt to talk someone into something. That is a power play.
- Sometimes people talk a lot for emotional reasons trying to justify what they want or are doing. Feelings of inadequacy create this kind of talking behavior.

Problems You Face Because You Talk a Lot:

- You are called a chatterbox and probably always have been.
- People say, "You don't listen" or "Get to the point." They get exasperated with you.
- Your spouse says, "Give it a rest" and tunes you out.

Your Goal:

To be in charge of your talking so that you are effectively heard, appreciated, and understood.

What Not To Do:

Do not ignore other people's reactions to you, but also know you deserve to be heard.

Your Work:

1. First you must notice if you are dominating conversations. Look at how much others say in contrast to what you say. Does the other person begin to form words, open his or her mouth, or start to say something as you talk right over him or her? Are you unable to stop talking until you finish what you have to say?

   I will begin to notice others' behavior instead of being un-aware of a person while I'm talking. _____yes

2. If a person snickers and rolls his or her eyes while talking with you, ask what the nonverbal expression means. These are signs that something is amiss. It may or may not be a re-sponse to your talking.

   On my way to finding out if I'm talking too much, I will ask others about their nonverbal communication while they are with me. _____yes

3. Make a note to stop talking right away when someone has something to say so you can learn to share conversation time. Even if you lose your train of thought, you are reaching for a more important goal—to learn to converse. In time, you will be able to both talk and listen without forgetting.

   I will break up what I have to say into short segments. _____yes

   I will pay attention to anyone I'm talking with
      so that I truly hear what they are saying and
      can respond.   _____yes

4. Before starting to talk, ask the other person, "How much time do you have to talk?" or "Are you on a deadline?" Also ask, "Do you have time for a story or shall I save it for later?" If the person is short on time, get right to the point without explanations or stories. Consider a situation where you can practice shared talking with another person.

   I can practice shared talking with _____
   when I see the person on (date) _____ .
   I will start by finding out how much time the
      person has for our conversation.   _____yes
   I will practice getting right to the point.   _____yes

5. After the shared talking, analyze your talking by asking some questions of yourself. Picture the conversation in your mind and ask the following.

Do I recall what the other person said to me?   _____yes

Do I feel I shared the time somewhat equally
between talking and listening?   _____yes

6. Congratulate yourself if you shared the time and can recall what the person said. You're learning.

I will write "I did a good job!" _____yes

7. Thinking again of the conversation, consider whether you tried to control the conversation to get what you want.

Did I press the person to do things by verbally
trying to convince him?   _____yes

Do I badger people into giving me what I want?   _____yes

8. Another reason you may try to control the conversation is to justify your actions to others. You may even be justifying your very existence. Though it feels bad to feel insecure, it's *your* job to learn to feel better about yourself, not theirs to make you feel better. So don't talk endlessly to everyone with whom you come in contact in order to feel adequate or valuable.

I do feel insecure.   _____yes

If I'm really honest with myself, I think I talk
too much in order to try to justify what I
have to say to others.   _____yes

9. Assume that anyone you're doing business with accepts you and your skill level. See yourself as a capable person. If you can't pull this one off on your own, see a counselor to help you.

I realize that people accept me and my skill level. _____yes
_____no

I feel doubtful about my value even though I think I come across okay to most people. _____yes

When I visualize myself as a capable person, I see _____

_____

_____.

10. If you've gotten yourself into a situation where someone doesn't value you and after talking with the person you still do not feel appreciated, consider finding a more compatible job or personal fit. That person is building his or her low self-esteem by using you. It's imperative that you not reinforce the negativity dumped on you.

I can think of someone who doesn't value spending time or working with me. That person is _____.

11. If there is more than one person, are they in a group? Sometimes peer pressure creates a scapegoat situation. You sure don't need to be used as a scapegoat.

    There is a whole group of people who seem to hang out together and I'm the odd person out. _____yes

12. Seriously look at leaving that setting. At least keep to yourself until you can figure out a way to find more compatible people to be with.

    I will leave the setting as soon as I can.   _____yes

    I will look for other people to spend time
       with and test out my conversational skills
       to be sure I'm not alienating others.   _____yes

    I can't leave the setting right now, but I will
       keep to myself so I don't get hurt and I'll
       focus on my job.   _____yes

13. Maybe everyone thought your talking was cute when you were young so it was reinforced. It no longer is, especially on the job where efficiency is important.

    I do have a history of chattering and used to
       get a lot of attention for it.   _____yes

    It no longer serves me well, however, so I
       want to get it under control and only use it
       when it is appropriate. I will work on this.   _____yes

14. If you have a serious low self-esteem issue or have always talked too much, you may have been trained growing up that you can get your needs met by talking too much. It could be that you talk others to exhaustion to get what you want. Or you may try to override what another person wants by wearing him or her down. These are power plays and do not belong in mutually respectful relationships. Stop it!

    I will stop using my talking as a power play.   _____yes

Your Commitments:

I commit to working on my talking.   _____yes

I commit to becoming a better listener.   _____yes

If I am unable to curb my talking, I will seek
   assistance from a professional.   _____yes

What Makes This Hard To Do:

Verbal habits and brain construction can add up to a lot of talking. You'll need to sort out how much of your talking is habit and how much is innate. Then commit to owning up to what you can change. You may never be a quiet person, but you can rein yourself in enough to be an enjoyable, if not delightful, person to be around.

Caution:

Incessant talking that does not yield to your conscious attempts to control it may be due to an imbalance in your brain chemistry that is called *obsessive talking*. If this is the case, you may be unable to control your talking without medical help. This is rare, however.

BLURTING THINGS OUT

Question:

Do you say things without thinking?

Why This Happens:

- The way you're made benefits you *and* causes you trouble. You are a keen observer, have a strong personality, and are very emotional. You also are likely to speak before you think. It's all part of your brainstyle.
- The more expressively dramatic and verbally active you are, the more you will tend to show your feelings and act upon them.
- But some of your behavior is the result of having been reinforced, even in a negative way, for your outbursts. And the reinforcement has probably been going on for a long time. Or maybe you've been trying to change someone's behavior by telling them what to do.
- You undoubtedly have an expressive nature, but if you haven't found appropriate channels for your expression, the inner need to discharge your talents will override your social judgment.
- As you have gotten older, part of your identity is tied as much to what you do wrong as what you do right. If you were not able to get things right early on, you, like all people, will tend to automatically go to the opposite extreme of being the most outrageous person you can be.

Problems You Face Because You Blurt Things Out:

- You shock people with what you say, forgetting about the values of those you're speaking with.
- You tell the truth when a little political savvy would stand you in much better stead, such as with the boss.
- By saying what you think, you hurt someone's feelings.

Your Goal:

To learn to use your strong opinions and skillful verbal potential in ways that clearly express who you are and get you self-esteem-enhancing attention.

What Not To Do:

Do not continue to act in a way that doesn't serve you.

Your Work:

1. List your observational skills.
   Are you quick to size up a situation?   _____yes
   Do you tend to see the truth under
      surface charades?   _____yes
2. List your expressive skills.
   Are you good with words?   _____yes
   Are you good with expressions?   _____yes
   Are you good with gestures?   _____yes
   Are you funny?   _____yes
   Are you quick-witted?   _____yes
   Do people find you entertaining?   _____yes
   Are you a natural storyteller?   _____yes
3. Ask yourself if you have a strong belief system. Do you stick
   with it when you are in the minority?
   I have a strong belief system and I do stick with it. _____yes
4. Once you've finished an assessment of your assets, look at
   your inner feelings of self-confidence and self-esteem. Do you
   find a difference between your talents and your inner feelings? If so, the discrepancy probably comes because you've
   developed your skills as an adult, but your feelings stem from
   when you were young and much more susceptible to others'
   judgments.
   There is a difference between my talents and my inner feelings about them. _____yes.
   I recall times when I was young when others' judged what I
   did and it hurt my self-esteem. _____
   _____
5. Ask yourself if you have been continually reinforced, positively or negatively, for blurting out things that amaze others
   and end up embarrassing you.
   I can think of a time when I was positively reinforced for
   blurting something out. It was _____
   _____ .
   I can think of a time when I was negatively reinforced for
   blurting something out. It was _____
   _____ .

6. Sometimes there is a particular person in your life who has made a big deal of your blurting things out. Do you think that was helpful or hurtful to you?

   _____helpful _____hurtful

   Maybe it was "their thing," which means it was not in your best interest. If this sounds familiar, write about it.

   I recall _____ making a big deal of my blurting things out. I can see an example clearly and describe it. _____

   _____

7. When you're ready, have a mental dialogue with that person, saying, "I know you haven't understood or been able to respond constructively to me. I'm now taking over the job of being in charge of my behavior, including my mouth. I appreciate what you've tried to do, and I forgive both of us for what didn't work. Neither of us understood that I could eventually learn to effectively take charge of myself, including my mouth, and let you take charge of yourself." Write this or something similar below if it fits.

   _____

   _____

   _____

   _____

8. Now think and feel about how you want to be. Ask yourself how you would like to express yourself. In what settings would you like to be dramatic? Then consider taking up theater arts work, improvisational activities, or public speaking. You can speak your piece that way and be rewarded instead of criticized.

   This sounds good to me. _____yes

   If you'd like to speak out on social issues, do so. Become verbal for a cause.

   I'd like that. _____yes

   Maybe you have an interest in motivating others.

   I'd like that. _____yes

   You could even become a radio personality, teacher, or counselor.

   I'd like to become:

   _____a radio personality _____a teacher _____a counselor

   But whatever direction you take, know that the very mouth that has gotten you in trouble can be used for constructive purposes now.

9. Once you've opened the door for effective self-expression, you can begin to work on keeping your mouth shut when you choose. Look at listening as a skill that will provide you with information.

I like the idea of learning to listen as a way to obtain information. _____yes

10. Store what you hear for later use. Make notes as soon as possible about what you censored coming from your mouth. These words will provide great fodder for future speaking, writing, and storytelling.

What I didn't say: _____

_____

I will use my words _____.

11. Once you've begun to learn to be quiet and listen, assess situations in which you find yourself. Ask what others need. What is their worldview? What do they value? How much can they handle? You have become a researcher by using these questions as guidelines. Choose a specific situation to observe and make notes about what you saw.

When I paid attention to _____,

I saw _____

_____

_____

_____.

Your Commitments:

I commit to use my gift of speech for my own benefit
and for the benefit of others.   _____yes

I commit to stay in control of my voice so that I do
not hurt others or embarrass myself.   _____yes

What Makes This Hard To Do:

If you have a long history of seeing yourself as an impulsive speaker, you are likely to feel helpless about changing. Though you may feel as if you face a daunting task, you can reshape your talking one step at a time.

TAKING ON TOO MUCH

Question:

Do you get in over your head by overcommitting?

Why This Happens:
- First of all, you undoubtedly have an enormously high level of physical energy. That simply means that you're constructed in a way that supports your engaging in many tasks without collapsing.
- The way your brain is constructed lends itself to multitasking.
- Add in your personality style that makes you a "helper type"—one who feels the need to respond to other people's needs—and you'll find it hard to turn requests down.
- You are likely to be sensitive, which is part of the reason you are aware of others' needs. If you're also kinesthetic, another aspect of that sensitivity means you'll want *to do something to fix* the discomfort created by a need you see. So you act *to fix* whatever presents itself as much for yourself as for the other person.
- Taking on so many things at once probably also means you have a brainstyle that predisposes you to become totally immersed in each thing you're doing as if it is the only thing you're doing. You tend to forget there are several of these "total immersion" activities going on at the same time. While you're engaged in one activity, it is the whole world to you. It's easy to forget when you are being asked to do something that you already said "yes" to a lot of other things.
- Occasionally, people do lots and lots in order to *prove* their worthiness. Though this explanation is often given, it is frequently not the real reason for overcommitting. More often there's nothing pathological about taking on a lot. It's more likely the way you perceive and experience your life events as they are shaped by your brainstyle.

Problems You Face Because of Taking on Too Much:
- You stress yourself with too much to do.
- You shortchange your family.

- You compromise your health.
- Occasionally a job doesn't get done as well as it needs to.

Your Goal:

To put yourself in control of what you choose to do so you can get quality as well as quantity out of your life.

What Not To Do:

Do not think there is something *wrong* with you because you do a lot, but also don't let yourself get so carried away that you short-change the special people in your life, including yourself.

Your Work:

1. Identify the different commitments, obligations, and projects in which you're currently engaged. Write them down below. Include activities with the family, paying jobs, hobbies, neighbors and friends, and community work.
   My commitments, obligations, and projects include:
   Family _____
   Paying jobs _____
   Hobbies _____
   Neighbors and friends _____
   Community work _____
2. Now put the name of each project, commitment, or obligation on a separate sheet of paper.
3. Rank the categories in order of importance to you and place the papers in that order.
   Category 1) _____
   Category 2) _____
   Category 3) _____
   Category 4) _____
   Category 5) _____
   Divide the various tasks that you are doing according to the categories you've selected. You may find that you have two different hobbies, two ways you earn money, one family obligation (with another pending), two neighbors you help, and three community projects.

4. Write the individual projects under the headings you've already created. Each sheet will have the name of the category at the top. Under it you will list the different projects by name. One sheet might read *Neighbors* at the top. Under it you would write: Ken and Joe.

5. Then step back, having laid the papers out in front of you. Look at them for a few seconds.

6. Then shut your eyes and breathe deeply. Ask yourself, "What's really important to me?" You may want to get away by yourself to sort out your feelings about this question.
   As I think about what's important to me, I choose _____
   _____ .

7. Once you've become clear about your priorities at this time—not for the rest of your life, but for now—again look at the papers. Reassess the commitments you have made. Ask yourself:
   Do I still have the same priorities I had a short time earlier?
   _____yes _____no
   If I have answered "no," I will reorder my priorities. _____yes

8. Follow through on the ones you've said you will do, but don't add any more until you work out a limit for how much you realistically can do.
   I agree to not take on anything else until I work out how many I can realistically do. _____yes

9. Reassess the number of items under each category. Then ask yourself, "Am I overloaded in any of the categories?" "Do I need to eliminate something?" "Do I need to eliminate a whole category?" If you're overloaded, it's time to cut back.
   I will eliminate the following item(s) _____
   under Category _____.
   I will eliminate the following Category altogether. _____ .

10. The number of commitments is less important than how you feel about what you are doing. Psychologically and physically, you'll feel more drained by some events and projects than others. Your emotional reactions will tell you which to keep and what to change. Deep inside, you know when you need to eliminate something.
    Listen! You'll hear warning signs in your head that tell you to slow down. Maybe you hear, "I really shouldn't say I'll do it." "My wife will kill me for this." Maybe you feel

your stomach twist. Or perhaps you feel guilty for taking on another task. These are all signs that you are going too far. When I assess how I feel about my projects, I find these feelings: _____

_____ .

11. Maybe you fear that you'll never be able to do something you want to do if you say "no" now. This is a frequent reason people overload. This can be a strong fear, but it's unfounded. You can almost always reconnect with a desire later on. You don't have to do everything now.
I feel afraid that I'll never get to _____
if I don't do _____ now.
I understand that I can reconnect with my desire later on.
_____yes

12. Learn to say "no." You need to get in the habit of saying it. To buy time, never make your decisions immediately. Say, "Let me think about this, and I'll get back to you tomorrow." By doing this, you're forming a habit, one that will stand you in good stead in many ways throughout your life. The next time something comes along, I'll practice saying "no," unless, of course, I really, really want to do it. _____yes

13. Having bought time, you can review your commitments. Check to see if you have room for an additional task in the category in which it fits.
From here on out, I'll buy time to check my commitments before agreeing to take something on. _____yes

14. Acquire a "commitment buddy." This is someone who will listen to you talk through the potential addition of something to your schedule. This person won't make the decision for you, but will remind you that you tend to overload and will help you be strong in saying "no."
I will ask _____to be my commitment buddy.

15. When you tell someone "no" but would like to keep the door open for the future, you can say, "I can't let myself take this on now, but I'd like to consider it later."
I can think of a situation where I might want to say this.
_____yes _____no
If not, write down the words here to help you remember them when the time comes that you might want to use them.

_____

_____

16. People will respect you for this approach. Your family will appreciate your willingness to spend time with them, and you will be in control of your life.

I like the feelings of respect and appreciation I feel because I've gotten control of how I spend my time. _____yes

Your Commitments:

I commit to respect my time and not over-commit
 to others or let them down when I can't do a
 quality job because I am overloaded.   _____yes
I commit to protect myself from burnout.   _____yes
I congratulate myself for seeing that I maintain
 a balance in my life.   _____yes

What Makes This Hard To Do:

Probably the hardest part of working on overcommitment is the feeling you'll miss out on something. Always promise yourself that you'll get back to whatever you're putting aside. Things of importance will always hang around, and you can nurture them into reality whenever you wish.

ATTENDING TO R & R

Question:

Is it hard for you to find time for rest and relaxation (R & R)?

Why This Happens:

- Being a naturally active person, you know more about doing things than not doing things. Doing little or nothing may seem foreign to you.
- When your main focus of attention is on work and family, you undoubtedly have a full schedule. To make time for R & R takes planning. And if that's not your strong suit, you could easily skip much-needed break time.
- If you don't plan regularly for R & R, you are likely to put it off until you're exhausted. Then is not the best time to find pleasant fun things to do. For one thing, you have to catch up from your exhaustion before you can enjoy yourself.
- You may also remember that there were too many times growing up when you could not be as active as you liked. So being inactive feels bad now. Such painful memories can lead to doing whatever you can to dull that pain including drinking, using drugs, running away—things like that.

Problems You Face Trying to Attend to R & R:

- You worry that your work will disappear if you take off.
- You don't know what to do or how to have a good time if you take off.
- You do foolish things when you do take time off.
- You can't organize your work time well enough to find the time to take off.

Your Goal:

To be able to plan R & R into your life in a form that easily fits you, your lifestyle, and your brainstyle.

What Not To Do:

Do not ignore your need for R & R or wait until you're exhausted to do something about it.

Your Work:

1. To find the right way for you, you'll need to notice whether you do things better if they are formally scheduled into your calendar or are better left to an inner sense of when you need R & R.

   I think that I do better planning specific times to
      to R & R and schedule them on my calendar.   _____yes
   I think that I do better simply taking time when
      I *feel* I need it.   _____yes

2. Check to see if you can tune into your body's needs. Some people can. Others can't. If you can, note whether you have the freedom to manage your own schedule.

   I can feel my body's needs. _____yes

   If you answer, "yes," then ask yourself whether you have the freedom to manage your schedule.

   I _____do _____don't have the freedom to manage my own schedule.

   If I do, I will take time when I feel I need it. If I don't, I'll schedule it in on a regular basis.

3. Next, decide if you prefer getting your R & R regularly (like exercising three times a week) or intermittently (like taking a long weekend every couple of months or after you finish a big project). Do you prefer a lot of little breaks or a few longer ones?

   I like regular breaks for R & R.   _____yes
   I prefer to intermittently take several days every
      couple of months or after I finish a big project.   _____yes
   I prefer a lot of little breaks.   _____yes
   I prefer a few longer breaks.   _____yes
   I like to make use of both kinds.   _____yes

4. Note the difference between rest and recreation. Doing something different from what you normally do, even if it's active, can be as rehabilitating as sleeping or doing nothing.

   I like to do things that are active when I take time off from work, at least some of the time. _____yes
   Sometimes I like to do absolutely nothing. _____yes _____never

5. If you're having trouble keeping on track with your R & R, check to see if what you're doing fits you. Going to a gym makes some people feel great, while other feel awful as they pick up all kinds of excess energy from the environment. One

person will love golf, or running, or holing up for a weekend with a stack of videos, while another will hate it.

During my time off, I like to _____

_____

_____ .

During my time off, I am now doing _____

_____

_____ .

I am doing what I like to do on my time off. _____yes

6. Don't pay attention to what others say you *ought* to do. Do whatever you want as long as it's not illegal or harmful to your health or another person. Disregard anyone who doesn't understand the choices you make.

I feel guilty or that somehow there is something wrong with me because I don't like to do what others like to do on their time off. _____yes

There's someone in my life who says I *should* like to _____ on my time off. That person is _____ .

I agree to disregard that person's advice, telling them "Thank you for sharing what you like, but I prefer to do _____."

7. Just as cross-training helps keep some athletes' motivation high, so does doing a variety of activities work better for some people. Others like getting into a routine of doing the same thing all the time. Either is fine.

I like to engage in a variety of things including _____

_____ .

I prefer to do the same thing all the time, which is _____ .

Your Commitments:

I commit to honor my need for R & R.   _____yes
I commit to make sure I have the kind of R & R
   I like in my life.   _____yes

What Makes This Hard To Do:

Friends and relatives may have their own ideas about what R & R ought to look like. Often they make suggestions and say, "You ought to go do . . . ." They are really saying, "*I* like to do such and such" and so assume that you will like it too. Be kind. Say, "Thank you." And don't succumb to their influence if it doesn't fit you.

DEALING WITH DRUG OR ALCOHOL USAGE

Question:

Do you wonder whether your drug or alcohol treatment journey is identical to everybody else's?

Why This Happens:

- If you have been chronically under stress, pressured for as long as you can remember to do things that aren't a good fit for the way you're made, you are likely to want relief. Alcohol and "pot" are two of the more accessible ways to do that and are two typical drugs of choice by people with sensitive natures who find it hard to deal with situations that don't fit their brainstyle.
- Because of a lack of understanding of brain diversity, many people experience undue tension, anxiety, and depression daily. If you're like this, the stress disappears quickly when you learn ways to live day by day that fit your natural self.
- Drugs and alcohol medicate the secondary symptoms (see the introduction at the beginning of this book) that result from living in a society that does not understand and hinders the expression of your natural brainstyle.
- Twelve-step programs are designed for people with addictive personalities who need to continually work with their addictive tendencies. They also help people who are suffering emotional and chronic pain from wounding at an earlier time. Participants benefit from the support of others who have been down the road ahead of them. A constitutional addict does not lose the desire for drugs or alcohol by understanding brain construction or finding environments that fit. A psychologically wounded person doesn't lose the desire for drugs or alcohol by changing his or her environmental fit.
- If you're medicating yourself to relieve stress created by a mis-fitting environment *and* you're not constitutionally addictive, you will follow a different path to recovery. With information, environmental management, and the acquisition of skills that help you live according to your natural bent, you are likely to leave problems with chemical dependency behind.

Problems You Face Dealing With Drug or Alcohol Usage:

- Even though you're working with a program such as Alcoholics Anonymous, have quit drinking, and have learned a lot, you aren't getting the relief others in the program are getting.
- Your problems with organization and the stress of paperwork and details as well as your sensitivity makes you want some relief, which makes you susceptible to taking drugs or using alcohol to feel less stressed.
- You wonder if your drug and alcohol journey is different from some of the other people in your AA program.

Your Goal:

To cease drinking and using drugs *and* learn about the management of your particular style of brain construction.

What Not To Do:

Do not assume that everyone who uses drugs or drinks too much is chemically dependent for life. And do not use brain diversity as an excuse to indulge.

Your Work:

1. No matter what, you must immediately cease drinking, if you are in any way dependent upon it or you have problems because of drinking. You must totally stop using drugs if they were your stress reliever. And you must listen to your addiction's sponsor, family, and friends who will tell you truthfully about any problems you have related to chemicals.
   I commit to immediately cease drinking if that
     is my drug of choice.   _____yes
   I commit to immediately stop using drugs.   _____yes
2. Begin to attend an AA (Alcoholics Anonymous), NA (Narcotics Anonymous), or CA (Cocaine Anonymous) support group and learn the principles of a twelve-step program. Work your program.
   I commit to immediately find the group that fits me and attend regularly, learning the twelve steps to recovery. _____yes
3. Next, it's important to learn more about your style of brain construction. All people are stressed when they are continually

thrown into situations that require a brainstyle that is different from theirs. People with a lot of ADD attributes are often stressed when they are trying to do jobs that require a lot of detail work, organization, and self-structuring.

I recognize that my brainstyle is _____linear, _____ADD, or _____ has traits of both styles.

(See *Attention Deficit Disorder in Adults*, fourth edition, for assessment guidelines to help you determine your brainstyle if you are unsure what yours is.)

4. Learn about managing daily living at work and at home based upon your style of brain construction. Learn multiple ways to relieve stress. Build a repertoire of skills that reflects your brainstyle.

I am learning to manage my daily living at work.   _____yes
To do this I am _____ .
I am learning to manage my daily living at home.   _____yes
To do this I am _____ .
I am learning to relieve stress other than by
    using chemicals.   _____yes
To do this I am _____ .

5. Read about creative and successful people with a brain construction similar to yours.

_____, _____, and _____ have brainstyles similar to mine. I will get familiar with their lives and what they do to make their lives work for them.

6. Learn meditation techniques and ways to get R & R that don't involve drugs or alcohol.

I like to _____ and commit to make it a part of my daily living. _____yes

7. Check the career/job/homemaking part of your life.

Does it fit me?   _____yes _____no
Am I being productive?   _____yes _____no
Am I being myself, doing what I
    love to do?   _____yes _____no
Am I glad (most of the time) to get up
    in the morning because I am pleased
    with my agenda for the day?   _____yes _____no

8. If your answer is "no" to many of these questions, then immediately begin to restructure your work life. Consider en-

gaging in career counseling that factors in brain diversity so you look at jobs that will fit you. Then make moves to change so you are in alignment with your potential and are able to use it more fully and satisfactorily.

I will read or study or get career counseling that takes my brainstyle into account so I can begin to plan to make changes that will allow me to use my potential and reduce stress in my life. _____ yes

9. Next, check your personal life. Be sure that you are in a mutually respectful relationship—one in which you and your partner work as a team. You each need to focus on one another's diversity and your respective assets, not your liabilities.

My personal life _____ is _____ is not with a partner who is respectful of me.

I _____ am _____ am not respectful of my partner.

We work as a team. _____ yes _____ no

We focus on our assets not our liabilities. _____ yes _____ no

10. Learn about diversity of brain construction in relation to household chores, entertainment, sex, and communication.

I will begin to do this. _____ yes

When? _____

11. Apply what you learn by looking at the world through your partner's eyes. This is hard, but do the best you can. It takes time and lots of talking, not arguing and not necessarily problem-solving, but sharing of perceptions with the emphasis on understanding and appreciating each other. Then, creatively find ways to meet both sets of needs.

Here's what I think my partner values:_____
_____
_____.

Check your thoughts with him or her.

I was right about what I thought he/she
    valued.   _____ yes _____ no

I will continue to have discussions with my partner to determine how we see things and then build ways to meet both of our needs, regardless of whether they are similar or different. _____ yes

12. As you attend a twelve-step program and come into alignment with your natural self, become aware of how similar and different you are to those around you.

I am similar to those around me in the following ways:

_____

_____

_____ .

I am different from those around me in the following ways:

_____

_____

_____ .

13. Be aware of how much or little you continue to struggle with a desire for alcohol or drugs after you've come to understand your brainstyle and have adjusted your life accordingly. Reduction of the stress from trying to live a life that doesn't fit your brainstyle may alleviate your desire for alcohol or drugs. On the other hand, you may still struggle because only part of your chemical dependency struggle was in relation to the pressures on you because of your brainstyle—one that didn't fit what you were doing. You may also have other issues and chemistry that makes you susceptible to chemical dependency and these must continue to be dealt with.

After changing my life to fit my brainstyle, I
     no longer feel a desire for drugs
     and/or alcohol.   _____yes
I still have a desire for drugs and/or alcohol
     after I changed my life to fit my brainstyle.   _____yes
Because I answered "yes" to the last question,
     I must continue to work my chemical
     dependency program and search for other
     issues that make me susceptible to addiction.   _____yes
I will continue to do this.   _____yes

14. Regardless of my brainstyle, I will stay alert to problem drinking or drug use and ask those close to me to do the same. Consider whether you were responding to a lack of awareness of what the True You needed to be effective and at peace. If you were trying to reduce the stress of an ill-fitting environment, put emphasis on being sure you honor your brainstyle and true nature. As a result, you may find you have no need for alcohol or drugs. But *be very careful here.* Don't fool yourself into thinking you can use alcohol or drugs when you can't. Use precaution and input from others in the program.

If I am considering that I do not, in fact, have an
   addiction to drugs or alcohol, I will carefully
   examine how I feel and act toward them.   ____yes

I will also get input from others in the program.   ____yes

I will err on the side of caution and continue
   to work my program indefinitely avoiding
   drugs altogether and considering the use of
   oalcohol nly after I am absolutely sure that
   I am no longer susceptible to its effects.   ____yes

I am prepared to immediately return to total
   abstinence and work with my program at any
   sign of vulnerability.   ____yes

Your Commitments:

I am committed to caution in sorting through the
   relationship between chemical dependency
   treatment and my brainstyle.   ____yes

I wish to honor my True Self.   ____yes

I will do nothing to compromise my True Self or my
   recovery from chemical dependency.   ____yes

I will remain alert and responsible as I sort through
   the relationship between my brainstyle and my
   problems with chemicals.   ____yes

I will seek input as I sort through the relationship.   ____yes

I will immediately seek help if I have any problems
   with drug or alcohol abuse.   ____yes

What Makes This Hard To Do:

Twelve-step programs have made an enormous contribution to all
people who have addictions that rule their lives. Yet not everyone
who becomes involved with alcohol or drugs requires ongoing dependency on a group for the rest of his or her life.

   This can be a scary thought for anyone who has struggled with
chemical use. You and those around you will know whether you
need continuous support of this type once you've honored your
True Self.

GETTING HIGH

Question:

Have you gotten into difficulty because of wanting the high that comes from things you do?

Why This Happens:

- You are likely to be an incredibly sensitive person who feels everything acutely. That means you can get devastatingly hurt and joyously happy.
- You live by your feelings more than your thinking. That's just how you are. Feelings provide you with information. You grow from them and you express through them.
- If you have a high energy level to boot (physically, mentally, or verbally), you will also tend to have a high level of volatile feelings.
- If you are kinesthetic, you will tend to act out your feelings.
- One thing that makes some people feel good is doing something exciting. So you begin with the excitement that comes with doing something that has a risk or pushes the limits. You feel great as a result. You express your great feelings by acting on them. Then you get even more excited. Thus a cycle of excitement reinforces itself, increasing your good feelings—and that's very psychologically addictive.
- Moderation is lost in the cycle of excitement. Your behavior can take on an addictive tone as you seek more and more excitement.
- Untrained in the rhythm of your brain construction, you have little hope of finding a moderate way to handle the enormity of feelings and stimulation by which you live.
- In addition, every time you feel down, bored, or stressed, you are likely to recall how good you felt when you were doing something exciting that made you feel high. The temptation becomes strong to repeat an activity that brought you the good feeling previously, so off you go, taking a risk to make yourself feel better.

Problems You Face Because of Getting High:

- A feeling of letdown follows getting high.
- You may even become depressed.
- The feeling of getting high doesn't really meet the need it's intended to meet and leaves you wanting.

Your Goal:

To seek outlets to achieve a high without hurting yourself until you build your skills to achieve moderation.

What Not To Do:

Do not let your feelings run rampant, and do not make promises that you'll "never seek excitement again."

Your Work:

1. Seek outlets to achieve a high that do not get you into trouble while you are working on building your skills to achieve moderation.

   I am willing to seek ways to achieve a high that won't hurt me or get me in trouble while I build my skills to achieve moderation. _____yes

2. Determine if you have a tendency to overdo and overindulge in activities that give you a high. To do this, ask yourself some questions.

   Do I overdo things? _____yes

   Make a list of these things, starting with when you were a kid.

   I overdo/overdid with _____

   _____ .

   Were you often told that you didn't know when to stop? _____yes

   Who said this? _____ .

   Do you smirk or feel like a "little dickens" who is getting away with something when you engage in an activity that excites you? _____yes

   Who said this? _____

   Do you feel as if you have to reach a high for relief or pleasure? _____yes

   What price have you had to pay for your overindulgence? Be strictly honest. List everything from scoldings as a child to confinement as an adult. Include loss of friends or jobs.

   Here's my list of what I've lost because of needing to get high on activities: _____

   _____ .

   Are you tempted to keep on doing some things that give you a high even though you have made other commitments?

   I am tempted to continue to seek a high. _____yes _____no

Can you walk away from something exciting without suffering or feeling torn?

I _____can _____cannot walk away from something that excites me without suffering or feeling torn.

When you are doing something that charges your emotions, can you let go of it for a time, knowing you can return to it at a later date?

I _____can _____cannot walk away for a time from something that charges my emotions.

3. Look at your answers and get a sense of how stressful it is for you to move in and out of activities that excite you. Rate yourself on a scale from one to ten, with one being "not at all" and ten being "unbelievably stressful."

I rate myself a _____.

4. Become not only aware of your feelings and needs but be aware of their effects in relation to another person. What is the effect on you and on other people in your life?

The effect on me is _____.

The effect on _____ is _____

_____ is _____

_____ is _____.

5. Begin to get familiar with the sensitivity that resides within you rather than immediately covering it with some form of activity that's accompanied by the enticing feeling a high brings.

I will do that. _____yes

6. Learn to protect and express your sensitivity in other ways than covering it with a high feeling. (See sections on temper control earlier in this chapter.)

I will do this. _____yes

7. Once you're clear on whether or not you have a problem being addicted to a high, commit to yourself that you will find ways to experience good feelings—highs—that won't hurt you or others.

I will commit to finding new ways to feel good. _____yes

8. Open new doorways through which your passionate nature can flow. The trick is to find things to do that are exciting *and* won't get you into trouble. For example, you can become an adventure writer or journalist who travels to the source of your stories for information, or you can work abroad. There's

mountaineering, rock climbing, acrobatic flying, race-car driving, deep-sea diving, and whitewater rafting. There's work as a firefighter, EMT, and undercover police officer. There's caving and skydiving.

For more sedentary people, there are activities such as playing the stock market or becoming involved in games that have risk and excitement. There's improvisational theater, stand-up comedy, talk radio, and investigative reporting. The list is endless.

Some of the things I might do either professionally or as a hobby include

_____

_____

_____ .

9. To get in control of your addiction to highs, don't bother to make a promise that things will be different next time or that you will settle down. That's unrealistic.

I will work at not being deluded that things will change *next* time. _____yes

10. Be sure that if you are in an intimate relationship with someone whose brain construction isn't like yours that you explain what you need.

On the one hand, a supportive person can enjoy your pleasure and encourage you. On the other hand, you can give the person permission to raise an eyebrow at you, if you begin to fool yourself or push reasonable limits too far.

I choose _____ to work with me on managing my highs in a constructive way.

11. But be cautious if you are constantly scolded for "how you are." You must simply "own" your own nature, holding up your end of being responsible for your activities. But don't let yourself be "tethered" to a traditional lifestyle that sucks you dry. If you do, you will tend to begin to sneak around and are more likely to get into some big trouble because you are not openly adjusting for your needs.

When I look at the people with whom I'm involved, I worry a bit about the lack of confidence in me by _____.

If I get a feeling that I might want to sneak around, I'd better look at what's prompting me to feel this way. _____yes

I wonder if someone in my life is too suffocating for my brainstyle. It could be _____ .
I commit to bring this out in the open and take responsibility for being who I am, acting in a healthy way while still expressing my True Self. _____yes

Your Commitments:

I commit to honor my brainstyle's urging to
   take risks within reason, engage in exciting,
   adventurous activities that fulfill my need.   _____yes
I will not, however, get out of control, letting my
   desires rule me.   _____yes
I will make sure that the price I and those around
   me pay for my interests and desires is not higher
   than is reasonable.   _____yes
And I will commit to work so that mutual
   understanding
   between me and those I care about allows each of
   us to do what we desire while not hurting the other.   _____yes

What Makes This Hard To Do:

Only you can ultimately be responsible for control of yourself despite the intensity of the urges within you. You must know when and how to ask for help. You must be responsible for when you get off track and protect yourself from your innate tendency to seek a high that gets out of control. You must stand by your True Self and not try to be anything you are not. You can do it!

OVERDOING ACTIVITIES

Question:

If you like something, do you usually find yourself doing it in excess?

Why This Happens:

- You are likely to be a person who tends to only be able to do one thing at a time. It's the way your brain works, sort of like you have an "On-Off" switch without a dimmer control to modulate the light. As a result, you tend to become absorbed in whatever you are doing to the exclusion of all else.
- Add to this your tendency to be someone who experiences life primarily through your sensitive feelings.
- You are likely to emotionally flood (See "Feeling Over-whelmed" in chapter 4)—be flooded with feelings and stimu-lation—so that you will experience an onslaught of emotion. As a result, when something feels good, it feels fantastically good.
- Also, if you are a person who does not readily break big proj-ects into small pieces, you may have difficulty finding your way step-by-step through anything you try to do. Instead, you dive in headfirst and grab onto whatever feels good. You cling to that until something else very important gets your attention.
- So here you are a sensitive, emotionally porous person with-out defined limits who has difficulty moving from one step to another. You feel everything intensely and are already proba-bly bruised by a world that is tough on people constructed like you. It's no wonder you revel in any good feeling that comes your way.

Problems You Face Because of Overdoing Activities:

- You get out of control, spending a lot more time with an ac-tivity than originally planned so that you shortchange your family and maybe even your work.
- You burn out from doing too much of a good thing, wasting the money you've invested in equipment, lessons, and other things associated with the activity.

Your Goal:

To find ways to use your intensity constructively while paying attention to the important people in your life and taking responsibility for your daily living.

What Not To Do:

Do not helplessly succumb to your behavior, overlooking others' needs and failing to live a responsible life.

Your Work:

1. In your pursuit of finding constructive ways to use your intensity while paying attention to the important people and responsibilities in your life, realize that you have a natural tendency to focus exclusively on one thing at a time. There's a good side and a bad side to this.
   I plan to reduce the negative side effects of a tendency to over-focus and increase the constructive use of those tendencies without getting out of control. _____yes

2. Your tendency to focus can seduce you to lose yourself in an activity. In the process, you lose track of time. Realize that when you lose track of time, you lose track of your life. You will need to take steps to be sure that is how you *want* to live your life.
   I commit to trying to be alert to those times when I lose track of time. _____yes

3. Revisit your value system. Ask yourself, "How do I want to live my life? How do I want to use my time?
   I want to live my life and spend my time in the following ways: _____
   _____
   _____ .

4. Make an assessment of your spiritual beliefs about *how* you choose to spend your time on Earth.
   I believe _____
   _____ .

5. Turn to your family and those about whom you care. Note their complaints.
   My family complains about these things that occur because of my over-focusing: _____
   _____ .

6. Ask yourself,

   Do I attempt to listen to the needs of those

      Iwith whom have a relationship?   _____yes

   Am I so focused on something that I don't

      hear what others say?   _____yes

7. Tell anyone you care about what you've been thinking. And tell the person that you want to change.

   Here's what I want to tell someone I care about: _____

   _____ .

   I will tell it to the following person/people: _____ ,

   _____, _____ .

8. Next, think about the time that you'd like to spend in your personal life. This includes simple things like eating dinner together, rocking the baby, playing with your child, doing chores, going on a date with your spouse, or, if you're single, spending time with someone you care about. You don't need to commit to all these things all the time. But start thinking about them and how much time you'd like to spend doing some of them every week.

   Some of the things that I would like to do because I've made more time in my personal life are _____

   _____

   _____ .

9. Ask your partner or friend what he or she would like to have in the way of involvement from you.

   When I asked about this, my partner/friend told me _____

   _____

   _____ .

10. Talk together, noting the times you both desire to make available for joint activities. Negotiate difference.

    We've come up with these times: _____, _____,

    _____ .

11. Next, you'll need some way to keep track of your time. If you're already using a day planner for work, you may want to continue to use it at home. Plot in time for your personal life and for any interests you wish to enjoy.

    I would like to use my day planner to schedule my personal life. _____yes _____no

    If not, how would you like to keep track of your time?

    I will keep track of my time by _____ .

12. Now it's time to discover if you are being enabled to maintain your intense interest in something at the expense of being

irresponsible to others on the job or in your family. Ask your-self, "Do others let me get away with shirking chores and jobs for which I need to be responsible while they fill in for me?" Do others enable me? _____yes _____no

13. If you answered "yes," turn to your enabler and share your new understanding. Own up to the fact that you've not been listening or committed to helping to fulfill his or her needs. Acknowledge you've not been taking on joint responsibility. Say you are now aware and planning to change. Ask the person to stop enabling you.
    I will meet with my enabler and also ask him or her to stop en-abling me. I will commit to be responsible. _____ yes _____ no
    If you answer "no," then you are not being enabled and you must carry the full responsibility for what you are doing. Tell the person directly that you aren't planning to change.

14. If you answered "yes" become specific. For example, if you pursue your activity past dinnertime, the family is to go ahead and eat. If you're still not present when dinner is over, the food is to be put away and you're on your own. And you don't get to leave dirty dishes in the sink after you finally eat.
    I agree to these guidelines. _____yes

15. You may need to rework your family budget if your activity is using a disproportionate amount of money. It's up to you to suggest making a new budget.
    I agree that I will bring up the idea of reworking the budget. I will do it by (date) _____.

16. Here's how to figure the budget.
    How much of your joint income is set aside for necessities such as housing, utilities, insurance, auto? Do not include extravagances like designer clothes or an extravagant car. These need to be paid for from discretionary income.
        $_____
    If you can agree, figure how much is to be set aside for future commitments such as your kids' education, retirement, investments.
        $_____
    Next, divide in half whatever is left over from the necessities and the savings for future expenses.
        $_____
    Each of you can do what you wish with this discretionary money. If you choose to use all of your discretionary income

for one activity, that's your business. But don't expect your spouse to cover for you when there's an opportunity to do something together that might be fun.

If you can't agree (even with counseling) on the amount of money to set aside for the future, you might divide the income after necessities as follows: Divide what's left into equal portions for each family member, including children. Theirs can go into their school fund or an investment to be used if something happens to you.

As a result, your partner may be investing for the future while you may not. The problem with this, of course, is that you won't be ready for the future when it comes. That time may seem far off, or you figure you'll have enough to make it up later. But it will probably put considerable pressure on your partner to turn his or her back on you if you are ever in need at a later date. This lack of responsibility for the future can put a terrible strain on the relationship. Remember, you must be responsible in the future for the choices you make now.

There is only one way to resolve monetary imbalances in a family because of one person spending exorbitant amounts of money on an activity: legally become separate. No matter how you handle money issues, it behooves you to face them squarely now.

I will face my money issues squarely now. _____yes _____no
If I choose to avoid them now, I will reconsider in _____ time.

17. Begin to help others who are like you to become aware of how you are constructed and what you're doing to help yourself. Show them how you are balancing a tendency to focus on one thing at a time while staying involved with your family and spending your time so it is thoughtfully under your control. You will be reinforced in your mastery by helping others.

I will help others with their over-focusing issues and, as a result, help myself. _____yes

Your Commitments:

I commit to work at getting control over my
over-focusing even though it may be difficult to do.   _____yes

I will recommit and take the reins of responsibility
   even though I've become lax for a time.
   I won't quit.   _____yes
I will also reach out to others to help them learn
   what I'm mastering.   _____yes

What Makes This Hard To Do:

Most people in today's world are looking for a magic cure—the "pill" or intervention that will change them. Instead, you must accept how you are constructed and live in the process of using your traits positively and responsibly.

4

Using and Protecting Your Sensitivity

As with so many attributes that are affected by your style of brain construction, your physical and emotional sensitivity has an up side and a down side. The True You benefits from its level of sensitivity by reflecting compassion, empathy, keen observational skills, and the ability to creatively express beyond the lines of orthodox definitions. Functioning outside the boundaries of traditional thinking depends upon the flexibility and responsiveness of your natural limits—limits shaped by your creative style of brain construction.

But the Wounded You will have been hurt because of your sensitivity as you failed to effectively protect yourself from unwanted intrusions: actions, thoughts, and feelings. You've learned that being told "Don't be so sensitive" is useless. You know you are as sensitive as your brainstyle dictates—not more and not less.

This section of *The New ADD in Adults Workbook* will help you honor your sensitivity so you can make quality use of it, while simultaneously learning how to protect your vulnerability. The Accommodating You will learn many skills to protect your sensitivity while allowing you to stay active in a potentially hurtful environment. As a result, you will be able to utilize the True You to its maximum potential as you protect the Wounded You from further hurt.

CATCHING ANOTHER'S FEELINGS

Question:

Are you an emotionally sensitive person whose moods shift easily?

Why This Happens:

- If you get around someone who is experiencing feelings that he or she is not aware of or isn't dealing with and your emotional boundaries are thin, you are likely to begin to take on that person's feelings. You "catch their feelings," much like you would catch someone's cold, only this is on an emotional level. This happens because your emotional boundaries are porous and another's feelings of anger, sadness, anxiety, and so on simply flow into you.
- Let's say you ask someone how she is and the response is, "I'm fine." But you get a funny feeling that she's not fine. You are at high risk to feel whatever that person is feeling but is not aware of or not acknowledging underneath the "I'm fine" comment. This is your empathy at work as you experience what she is not expressing.
- The reasons for a mood shift often go unnoticed by those insensitive to them.
- Sometimes mood shifts happen when something you see, hear, or otherwise sense reminds you of a past experience. You recognize the feeling attached to that experience, and it can quickly and strongly change your emotions.

Problems You Face Because of Your Sensitivity:

- Suddenly for no discernable reason, your mood shifts dramatically.
- You fear you may have an emotional *disorder*.
- You become depressed about being so sensitive.
- Others think you have a mental health condition.

Your Goal:

To become aware that there is a tangible reason for your mood shifts. You learn what to do about them.

What Not To Do:

Don't automatically think there is something *wrong* with you. And do not assume your mood shifted for no reason.

Your Work:

1. Realize that there are *real*, tangible reasons for any mood shifts you experience, even if they are not readily apparent to outside observers. You may even fail to notice the source of a mood shift because you've been taught that "You just have mood shifts because your chemistry is off."

   I realize that what I've been taught about
   my mood shifts may not be accurate.   _____yes

   I recognize that there are *real*, tangible reasons
   for shifts in mood that I experience.   _____yes

   I also see that outside observers may not
   perceive what I felt.   _____yes

2. To figure out what is behind your mood shift, pay attention to what you were doing and thinking right before your mood changed. A mood shift can come from something you were doing, someone you were around, or something you were thinking. A mood shift can be caught from outside of you or stimulated by an inner thought. Bring to mind the last time you had a negative mood shift.

   The last time my mood plummeted, I was _____
   _____
   _____ .

   I ask myself:
   Who was I with? _____
   _____ .

   Who was I around, even at a distance? _____
   _____ .

   What happened? _____
   _____ .

   What was I feeling? _____
   _____ .

   What was I thinking? _____
   _____ .

3. As you ask the questions, note the images that go through your mind, or bits of conversations that play in your head or

feelings that you get in your body. Add to the notes you
made above.

Though it may take a little doing to heighten your
awareness, you will discover that your memory banks
stored the trigger for your mood shift. All you have to do is
recoup the memory. It may come forth in a picture, word
phrase, or sensation.

4. Believe in what you think, feel, and see.
   I will seek the memories surrounding the event.   _____yes
   I will accept what I see, sense, or hear in my
      mind.   _____yes
   I trust my perceptions.   _____yes
5. If it is someone you know whom you think of, check and
   see if you often feel a certain way around that person.
   When I'm around _____, I often feel _____

   _____ .
6. If the way you are feeling is not a way you'd like to continue
   to feel, it's important to separate yourself from the other
   person's feelings.
   I am willing to separate myself from the other person's
   feelings.   _____yes
7. Keeping the other person in mind, you can say to yourself,
   "I pull my identification out of the situation." Or you may
   say, "I do not identify with so and so's feelings."
   I will say _____ .
8. Visualize yourself breaking the emotional connection that
   attaches you to that person's feeling as if you are cutting
   cords that tie you together to the person.
   I can visualize cutting the cords that connect us.   _____yes
9. Check to see if you begin to feel better. Your mood may
   even improve within minutes.
   I felt better.   _____yes
10. Arm yourself emotionally with a nonporous coating if you
    have to be around the person repeatedly. This could be vi-
    sualized as a coat of armor, distance, or a fabric that emo-
    tions can't penetrate.
    I see myself coated with _____ .

Your Commitments:

I commit to protect myself from feelings that don't
   belong to me.   _____yes

I commit to seeing myself as emotionally healthy
   even though I am sensitive to others' feelings.   _____yes

What Makes This Hard To Do:

Being susceptible to others' feelings and influences, because of your porous emotional boundaries, is a fairly new idea in this culture. Therefore, you may not find much understanding or support in what you're doing and how you're feeling. Even those you love may think there is something wrong with you. Professionals will often label you with an emotional problem that is called "biochemical," when really you are simply reflecting the effects of emotional energy that is coming your way unnoticed.

BEING SUGGESTIBLE

Question:

Do you catch the mood of the group in which you find yourself, sometimes to your disadvantage?

Why This Happens:

- Just as people vary in height, pain tolerance, or susceptibility to sunburn, so, too, do people vary in their emotional sensitivity to their environment.
- When your emotional boundaries are "thin," you will tend to react readily to the environment in which you find yourself. In a way, you *fuse* with it, becoming like it. That leads to your being suggestible as you're unduly influenced by what is going on around you.
- If you are a person whose feelings are more developed than your thinking, you will tend to be influenced in situations where you *know* better.

Problems You Face Because You're Suggestible:

- Your mood is dependent upon the mood of the group in which you find yourself.
- You can be influenced by the group or another person to do things that you wouldn't do if you were by yourself.

Your Goal:

To place you in control of your feelings and actions.

What Not To Do:

Do not allow yourself to get in trouble because of your suggestibility.

Your Work:

1. Recognize how you are naturally constructed, and do what you need to do to be in charge of your feelings and actions.
   I recognize that my brainstyle is _____,
   which makes me more susceptible to the influence of other people. _____yes

2. Accept the fact, in a nonjudgmental way, that you have a high level of sensitivity with less ability to self-protect emotionally than a lot of people. Acknowledge that you find it hard to "screen out" the emotional tone that surrounds you.

    I accept that I have a high level of sensitivity
        with a reduced ability to self-protect
        emotionally.   _____yes
    It is hard for me to "screen out" the
        emotional tone that surrounds me.   _____yes

3. Tell yourself that you are neither good nor bad because of the way your emotional boundaries are easily penetrated. Write this down.

_____

_____

4. Realize you can heighten your awareness about this and learn to get in charge.

    I can become more aware of my sensitivity
        and learn to get in charge of it.   _____yes
    I must guard against letting others influence
        my feelings and actions.   _____yes

5. When you enter a group, make a note about how you feel and what the tone of the group is. You may notice, for example, that there is a lot of frenzied energy. Or maybe individuals in the group are angry. Not all group energy is negative. You may move into an environment that feels peaceful and calm, and it will help you become peaceful and calm. Think of the last time you were with a group.

    The last time I was with a group was _____ .
    The tone of the group was _____ .
    I became _____ .

6. Consciously decide whether you want to let yourself pick up the energy of the group. Try this out the next time you are with a group of people or an emotionally expressive person.

    I was with _____ .
    I remembered to think about whether I
        wanted to pick up the energy of the group.   _____yes
    I decided to absorb the energy.   _____yes
    The result was _____ .

7. If you don't want to take on the energy of the group, visualize a barrier around you that keeps you emotionally separate.

Or you may want to imagine you are somewhere else that has the feeling tone you desire. Meditation will help you deal with the group. Stay alert and pay attention to your breathing.

I will try constructing a mental barrier around
      myself when I want to be emotionally
      separate.   _____yes

I will also give myself permission to leave a
      group any time I want.   _____yes

I've used meditation before and plan to continue
      to make use of it in this kind of situation.   _____yes

I will try out meditation if I've not used it before.   _____yes

8. Know that your heightened awareness can protect you, making up for your thin boundaries.

      My heightened awareness can protect me. I will write this now. _____

Your Commitments:

I will commit to learn to protect myself against the
      influence of others' emotional energy.   _____yes

I will construct an emotional barrier when I don't
      want to pick up energy that is negative or harmful. _____yes

I will use my sensitivity to reflect positive energy.   _____yes

What Makes This Hard To Do:

Not everyone is susceptible to the effects of his or her environment. As a result, others may not be able to empathize with you. They may even scold you or put you down because of your suggestibility. You will certainly be held responsible for it.

TAKING THINGS PERSONALLY

Question:

Do you tend to take things personally?

Why This Happens:

- Because of your inborn sensitivity, you feel everything keenly. That makes you extremely empathetic—a trait that yields compassion, caring, and openness to others. It also means you get your feelings hurt easily.
- Being someone who tends to look at the whole scene rather than the individual aspects of what's going on, you don't differentiate between what you are and are not responsible for. So, when something goes wrong, you take it personally.
- Because of your type of brain construction, you tend also to *become one* with everyone you meet. You become immersed in the person's attitude and demeanor. This means you take personally how others respond to you.
- Perhaps you haven't yet learned that it's okay to be naïve or ignorant or that there's nothing wrong with making a mistake.
- Your sensitive nature also makes you vulnerable to hurt from being scolded, chastised, shamed, judged, and emotionally attacked.
- You may not have learned to see another person as insensitive and boorish. Others have problems and feelings of their own that they are not taking responsibility for and, therefore, are unintentionally dumping on anyone who happens to be around.

Problems You Face Because of Taking Things Personally:

- You end up feeling depressed when people say or do things because they feel bad.
- You feel guilty and responsible when you did nothing wrong and no one meant to make you responsible.
- Your feelings get hurt very easily.

Your Goal:

To protect yourself from the hurt of taking everything personally.

What Not To Do:

Do not take everything personally that happens to and around you.

Your Work:

1. You must adjust for your natural style of brain construction so you are protected from the hurt of taking everything personally. I realize that my brainstyle makes me sensitive and that I take things personally. I will learn to adjust for this and not react. _____yes

2. Look honestly at yourself to determine how identified you become in what others say and do. Ask "What's happening here?" Think of a particular situation that happened recently. When I assess what happened around me so that I got feeling bad, I discover that _____
_____ .

3. When another person jumps on you, think through the situation so you can realize that the person may be stressed or feeling out of control. It probably has little to do with you. After all, people act that way when they are anxious, depressed, and angry even when they don't express these feelings clearly.
    I can recall a time when I jumped on someone else and it had little to do with what they did or didn't do and more to do with how I was feeling. _____
_____
    In retrospect, the last time someone seemed to glare at me or acted critical, they probably were feeling _____
_____

4. Don't bother to tell yourself to not take things personally. That's like telling your skin to not sunburn if you're fair complected.
    I will stop telling myself not to take things personally. _____yes
    I will also respond to others who tell me not to take things personally, "That's how I am. I'm working on it, but I am simply very sensitive." Or you may just shrug at their comment without verbally responding. _____yes

5. Engage your thinking and separate out your feelings for a moment. Ask yourself, "What more could I have done to make the outcome better?"

I could have _____

_____ .

6. Know you have choices. You can stop any transaction or situation that is uncomfortable and walk out. You can ignore a look or simply ask the person, "Are you having a bad day?" Only turn the tables if you feel strong enough to deal with this obviously stressed person. If you don't, walk away, knowing that you can always become supportive of others when you feel strong within yourself. Take care of yourself first.

I understand that I have choices. _____yes

I will listen to my needs and then determine
    how I want to respond. _____yes

7. Either journal about your feelings or talk them out with a friend if you are feeling bad. Then let them go. See them flying away into the sky or mixing with the earth.

I prefer to handle my feelings by _____ .

8. If there is something you can change, do so the next time you encounter the situation . . .

I agree to change or at least question my reaction the next time I come upon a situation where I feel personally hurt.
_____yes

9. Later, if you would like to work more with your reaction, you can continue doing the following: Get a mental picture of yourself as a young child. No, you're not acting childish now. But there is a likelihood that in addition to being thin-skinned, you also reacted so strongly because you've had previous experiences that have left emotional memories from previous *wounds*. The Wounded You recognizes previously hurtful situations. You bumped into an old emotional bruise.

I think I would like to try working further with discovering additional roots to my sensitivity. _____yes

10. Self-nurture that wounded part. Let yourself know you will protect it. Talk to that wonderful part of you saying, "I'm sorry you were hurt. There, there, it'll be okay." Then add something like, "I'll take care of you now," as if you're talking to a young child. Continue saying, "We can get out of here now. Come on." Make up the words that you would like to use.

I will self-nurture myself and protect my vulnerable feelings by saying,

_____

_____ .

11. If you want to take one more step, you can look in your mind's eye at the person or persons who created the bruise in the first place. Ask yourself what that person needed. After all, people are hurtful because they need something and don't know another way to get it. It could be anything from his or her fear of failure to a need to control everything, which is also a reaction to the fear of being helpless and out of control.

    When I think of the person who wounded me in the first place, I sense that person felt _____

_____ .

12. Consider forgiving that person for not doing better originally. You can do this if you know that you won't let your vulnerable part be hurt again. You are now in charge.

    I would like to forgive that person.   _____yes

    I am not ready to forgive the person.   _____yes

Your Commitments:

I commit to use the skills that I have to get over
  being hurt and taking things personally.   _____yes
I commit to explore further the other person's
  perspective so that I gain more objectivity.   _____yes
I will take care of myself.   _____yes

What Makes This Hard To Do:

You aren't likely to be able to completely change taking things personally. But by becoming aware of how you are made, you can spare yourself continued hurt and pain.

DEFENDING THE UNDERDOG

Question:

Do you frequently find yourself defending the underdog?

Why This Happens:

- Your innate sensitivity means you are very, very empathetic. You hurt when other people hurt.
- It's possible that your own memories of having been hurt are stimulated when you're around a situation where someone or something is hurt or wronged. The Wounded You is touched.
- As a big-picture person you are likely to see others, even animals, as an important part of your life—kind of one big family.
- Sometimes you hurt so much that you have to do something to remedy the situation. After all, as a kinesthetic person, you will tend to "take action" when a cause demands it.
- Finally, your strong feelings mean you lead with your heart, not your head.

Problems You Face Because of Needing to Defend the Underdog:

- You hurt when others are taken advantage of.
- You experience not only your own problems and sorrows but also those of others.
- You may get in fights or other trouble on behalf of another.
- You may not make as much money as you could or spend as much time with your family as needed because of your need to defend others.
- You may lose a valuable relationship because of how you feel and believe.

Your Goal:

You need be sure that you are making the choices you are making because you believe in what you're doing rather than taking knee-jerk actions because of your sensitivity. You need to be clear what the cost of your defense of others is, including the effect on your personal relations, family, partner, and children.

What Not To Do:

Do not stop feeling or become dulled to the hurtful things in the world. Do not, however, let yourself drown in another person's problems.

Your Work:

1. Even though you feel first, do not automatically act upon those feelings. Let a little time pass before you act.
   I will practice stopping and thinking before I act.   _____yes
2. Become aware of what you're feeling and why. Realize you are likely to take on the feelings of another person because you are very empathetic. (See "Catching Another's Feelings" at the beginning of this chapter.) Visualize a recent situation when you became enmeshed in the situation of another. Once you have the situation clear in your mind, examine your feelings of empathy.
   I see the situation clearly in my mind. _____
   _____
   When I examine my feelings of empathy, they look like this:
   _____
   _____ .
3. Find ways to use your feelings to identify situations that are wrong.
   When I think about _____
   _____ I feel bad.
4. Next, analyze those feelings and begin to think about what might be the most efficient way to act. If you don't think first, you can run around using up a lot of time without making much headway. And that behavior all too easily leads to burnout. Then no one gains.
   Continuing to think about the situation in retrospect, I realize an efficient way to act might be _____
   _____
   _____ .
5. It can be very noble, even heroic, to put your own well-being on the line for another person. But, before you do, be sure that is the best move to make for both of you. After all, if you both drown, there's no one left to tell the tale. Think about the implications of what you do. Then do the most you can

for the other person while considering how much you want to jeopardize your own position.

Again, as I think about the situation, I look at the potential implications of what I would do. They might be _____

_____ .

6. You must be careful that you don't do anything for another person that the person can do for himself or herself. If you do, you enable that person to stay inadequate and dependent. And, ultimately, you're taking advantage of the person so you can look good or not deal with your own emotional issues.

When I look at past situations, I see where, from time to time, I enabled others. Here's how I did it: _____

_____ .

7. Try taking a crisis intervention course. Through it you can learn how to help others effectively. Such courses can be found through social service agencies, churches, and emergency management groups. Start asking around and you'll probably find one.

I found _____ .

8. Consider multiple options to help others. You can become involved personally by becoming a teacher, mentor, or protector. You can speak out for a cause. You can create an organization or plan a remedy for a situation. You can write about the problem or become a fund-raiser not only for the person or situation but for others facing the same issue.

I plan to look into these causes and groups: _____

_____ .

9. You must also learn to protect your sensitive feelings so you don't "burn out." For example, if you rescue animals, you might begin with one or two, but pretty soon have ten or twelve. You might volunteer at the animal shelter once a week, then twice a week. Next, you might begin to worry about all the poor animals on days when you're not there. Finally, you decide to quit your job and work with the animals five days a week and eventually start going in on weekends, too.

When you're dealing with a perennial problem, you have to realize you can't save the world. And you must set limits on the part you will play so you don't burn out, becoming totally ineffective.

I am in danger of "burning out" in the following situation:

_____

_____ .

I will examine my underlying motives before deciding how to handle my situation. _____yes

They are _____

_____

_____

_____ .

Having done this work, I have decided that I'll _____

_____ .

10. Limit your exposure to problems. This may mean limiting the amount of television you watch and the news stories you read.

    I agree I need to limit the exposure I have to problems.
    _____yes

Your Commitments:

I commit to discover the underlying emotions and
    motives behind my actions.   _____yes
I commit to only do for others what they can't do
    for themselves.   _____yes
I commit to take care of myself so I don't burn out.   _____yes

What Makes This Hard To Do:

It's very hard for sensitive, kinesthetic people to ignore hurt and injustice. It's hard to face the fact that each of us has limitations with regard to how much we can accomplish in a lifetime to make things right. Know what you can reasonably do. Do it. Then let go of the rest.

FEELING OVERWHELMED

Question:

Do you feel overwhelmed, nearing panic, in new and crowded situations?

Why This Happens:

- A common reason this happens is because of something called "flooding."
- You see the big picture first before noticing details.
- When the True You is extremely sensitive, you tend to deeply experience what you see, feel, hear, and sense, both physically and intuitively. Too much stimulation comes at you too fast.
- It takes time to see the patterns created by the new situation and to figure out how things are working.
- With a job to do, you are better able to focus your attention; but caught off guard or with an unclear role or direction, you encounter an unpleasant experience.

Problems You Face Because You Get Overwhelmed:

- You may feel confused, so much so that you can't think clearly.
- Fear and feelings of panic may make you physically incapable of moving or you may become agitated and feel as if you want to run.
- You may become emotional, wanting to cry or scream, or you may become angry and hostile.

Your Goal:

You want to protect yourself from feeling overwhelmed when you encounter new and stimulating situations.

What Not To Do:

Do not press yourself or allow yourself to be bullied into prematurely moving into a new situation. Do not automatically think there is something pathologically wrong with you that requires medication and extensive therapy.

Your Work:

1. You can create an approach that fits you when encountering new and stimulating situations.
   I agree to create an approach that fits me when I encounter new and stimulating situations. _____yes

2. Visualize the last time you felt overwhelmed. Describe the setting.
   The setting was _____
   _____ .

3. Note what was going on around you. Asking the following questions may help you.
   Was there someone I knew there? _____yes
   What was the reason I was there? _____
   _____

4. Ask yourself what would have helped you.
   I would have been helped by _____
   _____ .

5. Having someone accompany you can make a big difference. That person can introduce you around.
   The next time I'm entering a new setting where I don't know people or what is going on, I'll see if I know anyone who is familiar with the group. _____yes

6. Even if you're alone, you can back up against the nearest wall, lean against it for support, and simply wait. Give yourself time to figure out what is going on. You'll either find someone you want to talk to, or something you want to do, or someone will come over to talk to you. That's the beginning. You're on your way.
   I will back up against a wall and wait until I figure out what's going on. _____yes

7. It's often helpful to have a job to do, something you planned out ahead of time. The more tangible the job, the better. For example, you may pass out brochures or appetizers, check people in, or help in the serving line.
   I would like to arrange to have a job to do the next time I'm in a situation that could overwhelm me. _____yes

8. Socializing in small groups can be helpful. Committees often work well to this end.
   I will attempt to be involved in smaller, more intimate groups both personally and professionally. _____yes

Your Commitments:

I commit to follow through with my plan to master
    situations I choose to be involved with.   _____yes
I commit to do what is in the best interest of myself.   _____yes

What Makes This Hard To Do:

Believing that everyone automatically knows what to do when entering a room or an event, you'll assume there is something wrong with you because you don't.

TAKING CHAOS OUT OF MEETINGS

Question:

Do you have a hard time knowing what is going on during meetings or gatherings?

Why This Happens:

- Because you have to figure out the patterns and processes involved, it will take you time to sort through the agendas at hand.
- You see the big picture, and that means there's a lot to look at all at once. Remember that many people who start something new don't see as broadly as you do. That is neither good nor bad. It just is.
- Besides having to figure out about the activity that brought you to the meeting, you are going to be inundated with everyone's feelings and personal agendas. This is because you are innately sensitive to everything around you.

Problems You Face in Meetings or Gatherings:

- You feel lost and confused in meetings and gatherings.
- You don't know what to do to get started.
- You wonder how others seem to know what to do even though they are new, too, and you feel you come up short when you compare yourself with them.

Your Goal:

To become comfortable and productive in meetings and gatherings.

What Not To Do:

Do not avoid groups.

Your Work:

1. Take your time adjusting to a new group. Study the people who are there. What roles do they seem to be playing? Look for group needs that are unfulfilled. Then notice where your skills might be needed. Think of a meeting you attended re-

cently or take these steps when you attend one that is coming up. Begin to practice these steps.

When I enter a new group of people, I will study the people who are there. I will watch what they do to meet people and I will see what they do to become involved. I see they _____
_____ .

I notice that the following needs of the group are not being met: _____
_____ .

I can offer the following skills to help out: _____
_____ .

2. Think about why you're there and what *you* want to accomplish.

   I am attending the meeting in order to _____
   _____ .

3. Notice who has the power in the group. The leader may or may not have the power.

   I notice that the leader has the power.   _____yes
   I notice that someone else has the power.   _____yes
   It is _____ .

4. Pay attention to individuals to whom you are drawn.

   I am drawn to _____
   _____ .

5. Ask questions that come to your mind, drawing others out so you can find how the group works. You don't need to appear to be all-knowing. Generally, people feel good when they can be helpful to someone new.

   Some questions that I can ask are _____
   _____ .

6. Be willing to take on a small helper's job initially so you can gain more time to figure out all the various aspects of the group.

   I see that I could volunteer to _____
   _____ .

7. Know your talents are important. The group will need your skills whatever they are when you're ready to make your contributions. Should you get into a group where a person practices territoriality, back off until you find a way to use your talents without threatening that person. You're the new one so you'll have to figure out where you can fit. For example, let's say you have photographic talent but someone in

the group has been taking the photographs for some time. You quickly realize that the person covets that job and doesn't want to engage in teamwork.

I have these talents: _____

_____.

I _____do _____don't have competition for my skills.

If I find competition, I will back off until I can figure out a way not to threaten anyone in the group.   _____yes

8. If all else fails, start your own group and let everyone else fit into it. This can actually be a very creative thing to do. It's often more work, but it can be very fulfilling—besides, you get what you want.

I would like to start a group that fulfills the purpose of _____

_____.

Your Commitments:

I will open my mind to developing new social skills.   _____yes

I commit to use my thinking mind as well as my
   feelings to figure out how to maximize the use
   of a group.   _____yes

I commit to think positively about time spent in
   group activities.   _____yes

What Makes This Hard To Do:

Impatience and feelings that you should know what is happening will make it hard for you to enter a new group situation. You will eventually become an asset to the group as you see patterns in the initial chaos.

TRAVELING WITHOUT STRESS

Question:

Does it take you a while on vacations to figure out how to relax and have fun?

Why This Happens:

- Traveling means you must change from your regular routine. Changes take time and effort for everyone, but sensitive people feel the changes particularly keenly.
- Though you can get into the groove of traveling (moving and changing), you must find your own rhythm first and that takes time.
- Once you've "gotten in the groove," you can turn your attention to having fun. Pre-planned tours may not work well for you because your adventurous self will want to guide you to your own types of pleasure.
- You must listen to your feelings for this to work. And that means you have to pay attention to your feelings first.

Problems You Face Because of Traveling:

- Stress from the time it takes to learn about new situations.
- Confusion, disorientation, and discomfort in mass transit situations like airports and bus stations.
- Lack of individualization and creative traveling on pre-planned tours.
- Lack of structured plans to make good use of your time.

Your Goal:

To find travel plans and arrangements that fit your rhythm.

What Not To Do:

Do not put yourself in a situation that controls you so you lose touch with your natural rhythm.

Your Work:

1. Do take your time and find your own rhythm in whatever kind of vacation you choose to undertake.

I plan to tune into my personal physical and emotional rhythm. ____yes

2. There are several kinds of trips. The first is a spontaneous, self-directed adventure. The second follows a pre-planned agenda of your own making. The third follows a pre-set package that requires little or no planning by you.

Do I immediately have a preference for one of these?

_____yes _____no

Mark the one you are most drawn to with a "1," the second one with a "2," and the least interesting to you with a "3." If you absolutely don't want to try one of these, mark it with a "0."

Plan 1: _____Spontaneous, self-directed adventure.
Plan 2: _____Pre-planned agenda of my own making.
Plan 3: _____Pre-set package with little or no planning by me.

3. In Plan 1, you spontaneously take off and simply follow your nose. Perhaps you flip a coin. If it lands on heads, you turn left (in your car, motorcycle, bike, or on foot). If it lands on tails, you turn right. You go when you want to go and stop when you want to. If this sounds fun or even a little bit interesting, do it.

I _____do _____ do not like the idea of Plan 1.

4. If you do like the idea of Plan 1, prepare for a number of eventualities. Pack enough food in your vehicle to last a few days. Have several changes of clothes, but travel light. Take some camping gear or enough money to rent a place from time to time. Take good maps or get them along the way.

In addition to the items mentioned, I'd like to take _____
_____ .

I also have some idea where I'd like to end up, but I don't care how I get there. _____yes

5. Know ahead of time how long you can/will be gone. Simply turn around when you've used up half your time.

I imagine I'd like to be gone _____ days.
I believe I can get to _____
in that time.

6. Ask "locals" where the good places are to eat and where interesting activities are happening.

I will ask for advice from locals and people I already know who have been to the area in which I plan to travel._____yes

7. If you enjoy talking to people and like to hear their stories, talk to people along the way. Everyone has a story and lots of information.

I ____do _____don't like to talk to people.
I plan to find out about them and the region in which I find myself. _____yes
Or I'd like to spend my time _____ .

8. Take a journal, paints, camera, or whatever creative materials you like.
   I will take _____ .

9. Stay flexible, always willing to change your plans.
   Flexible it is. _____yes

10. In the second form of traveling, Plan 2, you follow a pre-planned agenda of your own making. Here, you have some reservations with deadlines for arrival and departure. You may want to have a friend who is more linear than you help you lay out the itinerary ahead of time. Also consider a traveling companion who has planning skills you don't have.
    I'd like to try this form of traveling. _____yes
    I would like to go to_____ .
    I would like to ask _____ to help me plan.
    I would like a traveling companion. ____yes

11. Plan a couple of extra days for "getting adjusted time." Do not push yourself initially.
    I will take my time and make room for adjustments in my time and rhythm. _____yes

12. Do not spend a lot of money right away until you know the options that are available to you.
    I will keep close control of my money before I see what is going to be available to me throughout the trip. Then I can decide what I want to spend money on. _____yes

13. You don't need to necessarily follow the regimen that most tourists who go to the area follow. You are likely to want to create a trip that spends more time in one place than most people do and then skip another "typical" tourist site.
    When I think about going to _____
    I know I would _____ .
    I will also ask locals for suggestions, saying the kinds of things I enjoy doing. _____yes

14. Talk to more than one person about your options.
    I will gather lots of information. _____yes

15. You may want to hire a guide initially to get an overview of the region so you know what your options are.
    I like the idea of a guide. _____yes

16. When you are in a crowded place, be willing to ask questions—lots of questions.

    I will ask questions when in new and crowded places so I don't waste a lot of time wandering around. _____yes

17. If you get nervous in new, busy places like depots, remember to breathe calmly and moderately deeply. Shut your eyes, and remember who you are and that you are simply a traveler at this time who is having an adventure. Stay in the present time rather than worrying about what you'll do next and next and next.

    I will practice my breathing right now as I conjure a picture in my mind of traveling to a place I'd like to visit on my journey. I will commit to take one step at a time. _____yes

18. If you prefer to make use of a totally pre-planned package, Plan 3, probably with a group, spend time going over the itinerary beforehand. Check to see if there is anywhere along the way that you would really like to visit, stay longer, or deviate from the pre-planned itinerary. See if you can make arrangements before you leave.

    I am considering going to _____ with _____ group.

    I will check the plan and see if I would like to take a side trip. I would like to go to _____.

    I will check out the possibility ahead of time by contacting

    _____

    _____.

19. You also will want to do some investigating ahead of time to see who your traveling companions will be. Ask yourself if you have interests in common. How good are you around a lot of different people's energy? Do you have idiosyncratic timing, such as liking to stay up late at night and to arise late in the morning? Do you have special dietary needs?

    The group will consist of _____.

    I _____ do _____ don't have trouble around other people's energy.

20. If you do, consider whether you feel strong enough to protect yourself from a lot of energy outside of yourself or if you need to reconsider going on a group tour.

    I do feel a lot of energy from other people when we are in close proximity. Maybe I need to reconsider the trip I'm planning. _____yes

I _____ do have special dietary or sleep needs. They are
_____
_____ .

21. Remember that the point is to have a good time. And only
you can determine how you will fulfill that agenda by doing
what you want.
I will keep track of how I'm feeling and make sure that I am
doing what I really *want* to be doing while I'm traveling.
_____yes

22. If you're traveling with someone with whom you're not
compatible, you will probably be frustrated. Seriously consider splitting up for a while so you can each do what you
like. It's no one's fault. You just don't make good traveling
companions.
I've had that experience and if it happens again, I'll commit
to separate in both our best interests. _____yes

Your Commitments:

I commit to take the time before I leave on a trip to
tune into what I want to get out of this travel time.   _____yes
I will do what I want to do, not what someone else
thinks I would like or ought to do.   _____yes
I will not remain in a situation that makes me feel
emotionally down or hurts another person.   _____yes

What Makes This Hard To Do:

If you try to do too much in one trip, you'll overload yourself. If you
turn your power over to someone else and begin to do things you
don't want to do, you will begin to feel bad. Take your power back.

If you believe that trips and vacations are always wonderful and
never fraught with problems, you are likely to be disappointed.
Take interest in all that happens at the time it's happening instead
of over-focusing on the goal.

INTERRUPTING CONVERSATIONS

Question:

Do you find yourself "getting into trouble" because you don't mind your own business?

Why This Happens:

- Common reasons why you do not exercise the boundaries and limits others seem to see are because you focus more on the content of what is happening than the details. You probably focus more on the question than on a detail like who the question was addressed to. A person with a more linear style of brain construction is likely to see the situation in the opposite way.
- You may also have feelings of inadequacy and be trying to prove to others and yourself that you are knowledgeable.

Problems You Face Because You Interrupt Conversations:

- You get embarrassed.
- Others don't like the interruption.
- You may be told to "mind your own business."

Your Goal:

To recognize other people's business and act in a respectful manner, waiting your turn.

What Not To Do:

Don't interrupt and take responsibility for what hasn't been asked of you.

Your Work:

1. Learn to recognize other people's business and ask yourself if you think it's wise to cross into their turf.
   I am willing to learn respect for other's conversations and business. _____yes
2. Heighten your awareness. Right now commit to paying attention to how you act around other people. Do you butt in?

Do you override what they are saying? Do you offer advice when it's not requested?

I commit to paying attention to how I act
   around other people.   _____yes
I'll take time to observe my behavior in
   relation to others starting now.   _____yes

3. Ask yourself and observe whether you cut people off or intrude in their business.

Do I butt in?   _____yes
Do I override other people's conversations?   _____yes
Do I offer advice when I've been not asked
   to do so?   _____yes

4. Be honest with yourself. It may take time, but you'll get the knack of facing up to your nonproductive habits.

I commit to being honest with myself even though it may be painful.   _____yes

5. Focus on the people around you.

Here are some of the people close to me that I will practice on: _____
_____.

6. If someone asks a question, ask yourself, "Who spoke? Did that person address the question to me?" This is a critical step to learn to take.

When I ask myself these questions, I find that I _____
_____.

7. You are likely to feel guilty if you discover you interrupt frequently. But forgive yourself. You will learn new ways.

I feel _____ about my behavior.
I do forgive myself, however. _____yes

8. Observe if the person asked is quiet because he or she is thinking. Realize that people problem-solve at different rates. You may be able to come up with answers at lightning speed. But if another person can't, don't jump in prematurely, speaking for him or her. Consider the people you know. Make a list of those who are as fast as you. Then make a list of those who process information and conversations at a pace different from yours.

Those who are fast like me are: _____,
_____, and _____.
Those who process at a different speed are: _____,
_____, and _____.

9. If a person doesn't know the answer, you may then, and only then, *ask* if input from you would be welcomed. You need permission to join the conversation if you are not already a part of it.

    I commit to begin asking if my input is
      welcomed.   _____yes
    I will ask if I may join a conversation.   _____yes

10. Don't push the situation if the people involved ignore you or change the subject. Remember, this wasn't your situation in the beginning and you can only join in if you're invited.

    I will back off if I'm ignored or there is not an easy invitation.
                                                            _____yes

11. If you have feelings of inadequacy, check to see if you are trying to impress someone with what you know or are trying to prove to yourself that you're smart.

    I do feel inadequate. _____yes
    I feel I need to impress _____. _____yes
    I want to impress _____. _____yes

12. Check for feelings of inadequacy by sensing whether you are feeling uneasy in your stomach or are lightheaded. Note how your emotions feel. Are you afraid that you'll never amount to anything? Do you feel depressed because you feel you're not as smart as other people?

    Physically, I feel _____ when I'm around other people and want to be a part of what's going on.
    Emotionally, I feel _____ when I'm around other people and want to be a part of what's going on.

13. Realize that you learned these thoughts and feelings of inadequacy in error. The thoughts are untrue. You are not inadequate.

    I recall when I began to feel inadequate. But I know now that I'm neither inadequate nor potentially bad company. I will change the way I perceive myself, seeing myself in a brighter, better light. _____yes

14. Visualize yourself when you were younger and talk to yourself as a good parent would reassure a small child. Be a good self-parent to yourself.

    I see myself as a small child and can talk to her/him in the way that a good parent talks to a child who is loved and admired. I would say _____

    _____.

15. Tell yourself that you are a winner, as valuable and smart as anyone else.
I am _____
_____ .

16. Say "thank you" to yourself for being good to yourself.
I say, "thank you" _____ .

Your Commitments:

I commit to work on not interrupting others or trying
to mind their business. _____yes
I commit to being a good parent to my inadequate-
feeling self. _____yes
I congratulate myself on connecting to the True Me. _____yes

What Makes This Hard To Do:

Habits are hard to break. But remember, this is your first day committed to changing the habit of stepping into other people's territory. You can do it. Just take one step at a time. It doesn't matter if you don't do it overnight.

BORROWING WITHOUT PERMISSION

Question:

Do you sometimes get into trouble borrowing things without permission?

Why This Happens:

- With your eye on the goal, you forget the steps needed to reach it. Attention to the big picture does you in as you fail to see or acknowledge the details—details others consider important. In this case, your goal may be to get something done at work or dress well for an occasion. The steps you need to take include your asking "Who 'owns' the article I need to reach my goal?"
- Because you're a kinesthetic person, one whose action skills are highly developed, you may forget that an action that intrudes on another's turf crosses that person's physical boundaries.
- Tools, clothes, and all kinds of items belong to their owner, not you. In a culture that has strong guidelines for ownership, crossing these boundaries is considered impolite and wrong.
- If you feel emotionally close to another person, you may assume that what belongs to that person is automatically available to you and the person won't mind your *borrowing* it. You probably wouldn't mind if the tables were turned so you can't imagine their minding. Thinking this way means you experience things globally. By definition, seeing things globally automatically means you see them without limits and boundaries. So you may simply not see limits that others see.

Problems You Face Because You Borrow Things Without Permission:

- Others get angry with you.
- You aren't considered a team player.

Your Goal:

To not ignore physical boundaries, taking what doesn't belong to you without branding yourself a bad person.

What Not To Do:

Do not continue to ignore physical boundaries, taking what doesn't officially belong to you. But do not consider yourself to be a bad person either.

Your Work:

1. Learn how to control the global tendencies that are so much a part of you so you can use them when and where they are appropriate and restrain them when necessary.
   I would like to learn this. _____yes

2. Immediately realize that you can get in big trouble socially and even legally if you take what doesn't belong to you.
   Though I may not have considered the possibility, I now realize that I could get into big trouble because of taking something that doesn't belong to me. _____yes

3. When you want something, stop and think what individual steps are needed for you to get what you want.
   I can visualize wanting something, but before I make the move to "borrow" or take it, I stop. _____yes

4. Then see yourself stopping. Say, "Stop!" Replay this vision, immediately. From time to time, replay it.
   I will replay the vision from time to time. _____yes

5. Once you've said "Stop" to yourself, take the time to consider what individual steps are needed for you to get what you want.
   I continue my vision. I see myself taking the time to consider what steps I need to take, such as asking for permission from the person I wish to borrow from. _____yes

6. Practice looking around your workspace and through your personal belongings to note what belongs to you. Notice what belongs to others. This will begin to create two categories in your mind: "Mine" and "Others."
   When I look around at the things in my possession, I notice that some belong to other people. I will take an inventory of what is "Mine" and what belong to "Others." _____yes

7. Either return anything that is not yours or reaffirm your use of it with the person.
   I will immediately agree to speak with the person from whom I borrowed/took the item. _____yes

8. Make a habit of respectfully asking to use things that belong to someone else, even if that person is a family member or close friend whom you're sure won't mind. It's just good practice.

   I will ask any person, even a family member or close friend, when I'd like to borrow something. _____yes

Your Commitments:

I commit to be respectful of others' things.   _____yes
I commit to communicate with other people,
   even family and friends, when I want to
   borrow something.   _____yes

What Makes This Hard To Do:

Lack of awareness is probably the biggest obstacle you face in implementing a willingness to respect what belongs to others. Fortunately this is something you can work on.

RESPECTING JOB BOUNDARIES

Question:

Do you irritate people at work by mixing into their business?

Why This Happens:

- In reality you are likely to be very responsible. But if you focus on the goal of accomplishing the job that is given you rather than on *how* it is to be done, or who has the power with respect to various aspects of the project, you are likely to step on someone's toes, alienating coworkers.
- You may forget when you don't have responsibility for a project that you have no inherent right to make decisions that affect another person. Neither do you have the right to use something they have been working on unless they offer it to you.
- Anyone who pays more attention to details than the process of getting something done will likely get upset when you overlook the boundaries between what they're responsible for and what you are responsible for.

Problems You Face Because of Ignoring Job Boundaries:

- You may incur the wrath of coworkers.
- You may not be seen as a team player.
- You are viewed as disrespectful.

Your Goal:

Know the limits of your job and the tolerance of your coworkers for crossing those limits.

What Not To Do:

Remember that not everyone is constructed the way you are. Some are very serious and territorial about their work areas, ideas, and skills.

Your Work:

1. Know the limits of your job and the tolerance of your coworkers for crossing those limits.
2. Make a list of those who work immediately around you from whom you may "borrow." Then rate their tolerance for being

"borrowed" from 1 = not tolerant at all to 10 = extremely tolerant.

My immediate coworkers   Their tolerance level

_____   _____

_____   _____

_____   _____

_____   _____

_____   _____

_____   _____

3. Know clearly what assignment or job you're fulfilling and who's in charge. That will give you information about who has the power in any situation.

My job assignment is _____

_____ .

The person in charge is _____ .

4. Observe how flexible individuals are. Notice whether the organization reinforces shared work versus expecting each person to do his or her own task, or even reinforces competition.

The organization ____does ____does not
   support shared work.   ____yes
The organization expects each person to do
   his or her own work.   ____yes
The organization reinforces competition.   ____yes

5. Discover how territorial your coworkers are. Ask yourself how much they guard what they are responsible for. This could be anything from materials to space to ideas.

   Returning to the list of coworkers under #2 above, rate your coworkers on territoriality: 1 = not very territorial and a 10 means very territorial. Also note what they are territorial in relation to (e.g. materials, space, and/or ideas).

6. Ask before borrowing things, assignments, or time from a coworker.

I agree to ask my coworker if I may borrow from her
   or him. ____yes

Also ask before giving something that is not yours to another department or person. This includes little things like phone numbers and thoughts.

I agree to ask my coworker about lending something that is his or hers. ____yes

7. Be sensitive to others' responses to your offers to lend ideas, equipment, or time. Not everyone sees your generosity as

valuable. Don't push yourself on someone. Read their lack of response as an indicator that they are probably not interested in your offer but don't know how to say no.

I will become aware of others' responses to
any offer I make.   _____yes
I will not push myself on someone.   _____yes

8. Give anyone from whom you borrow acknowledgment for the role he or she plays in the final creation or project.
I will give anyone from whom I borrow both personal and public acknowledgment of their role in the final creation or project. _____yes

9. If you are extremely creative and carry a big vision of what-ever you do, you might want to consider self-employment, where you are the one in charge. That way you can put things together in unique combinations. You're free to do this as much as you like with your own business.

Or you may choose to look for a creative partnership or group that is clearly open to working in a boundary-hopping style.

Your Commitments:

I commit to raise my level of awareness of what is
mine and what belongs to others.   _____yes
I commit to respect the desires and territory of
others regardless of how I like things to be.   _____yes
I commit to be good to myself, placing my work
habits and desires in an environment that
fulfills me.   _____yes

What Makes This Hard To Do:

You may get focused exclusively on the process of reaching your goal, caught up as you are in the creative process. Or you may feel angry that other people "get in the way" of what you consider most important.

HUGGING AND TOUCHING OTHERS

Question:

Do other people sometimes pull away because you are more physically expressive than they are?

Why This Happens:

- As an expressive, kinesthetic person whose exuberant feelings abound, you may forget or even be unaware that not everyone is comfortable with the way you naturally express yourself.
- You may feel that another person's hesitation means they don't like you. But that is not necessarily true. Taking other people's responses personally is due to the way you see the world. (See "Taking Things Personally" earlier in this chapter.)
- Not everyone likes the same kind of touch. Being extremely physically sensitive, you and others may have distinct preferences for how you are touched and what touches your skin. Brain construction dictates these levels of sensitivity.
- You may be accused of being insensitive of other's feelings when, in reality, you may have only learned to ignore feelings altogether.
- Often, very sensitive babies and children are innocently hurt—even the roughness of fabric or the tags on clothes hurt. Those experiences can teach a child to disregard his own and others' physical nature.
- Not everyone shows his friendliness physically.

Problems You Face Because of Hugging and Touching Others:

- Others may stiffen or pull away from you, feeling uncomfortable.

Your Goal:

Learn to express your friendliness while taking another person's preferences into account.

What Not To Do:

Do not ignore another's reactions to you.

Your Work:

1. Right now, think about the people you know. Rank them according to how much you think each likes being hugged or touched. This may range from "Not at all" (1) to "Lots"(5). Place the rating number immediately after the person's name. I can think of the following people whom I'd like to rate:

    _____, _____,
    _____, _____,
    _____, _____,
    _____, _____.

2. Check with a few of the people with whom you have a close relationship about how they feel about touch. Also ask their opinion about people you know in common. This will help you develop sensitivity to other people's preferences.

    When I checked with _____, he/she said
    _____.
    When I checked with _____, he/she said
    _____.
    When I checked with _____, he/she said
    _____.

3. When you like someone, begin to ask yourself whether you think that person would like to be hugged or touched.

    I think _____ _____would _____would not like to be hugged or touched.
    I think _____ _____would _____would not like to be hugged or touched.
    I think _____ _____would _____would not like to be hugged or touched.

4. Begin to read body language. Consider the people listed in #3. Ask yourself the following about each one:

    Does the person pull away from me or lean toward me when I'm talking?

    _____ _____pulls away _____leans toward
    _____ _____pulls away _____leans toward
    _____ _____pulls away _____leans toward

    Does the person talk only about *things* or does he or she also talk about feelings and how he or she feels?

    _____ _____only things _____feelings
    _____ _____only things _____feelings
    _____ _____only things _____feelings

Does the person seem like an emotionally warm person or a cool one?

_____ _____warm _____cool
_____ _____warm _____cool
_____ _____warm _____cool

Does the person make eye contact with you?

_____ _____yes
_____ _____yes
_____ _____yes

5. If you're unsure whether a person will like being touched or hugged, ask, "Do you like hugs?" Notice whether the person reaches toward you enthusiastically or pulls back or looks restrained. Respect the answer. Never push.

   I will respect another's preference for being hugged
      or touched.   _____yes

6. If you are keenly sensitive to another's energy, simply stop and ask yourself how you sense the person. Then trust what you sense.

   I trust my sensitivity.   _____yes _____no

7. If you answered "no," what will it take to help you trust your sensitive feelings?

   To trust my feelings, it will take _____
   _____ .

8. Become aware of your own sensitivity to touch and clearly distinguish what you like and dislike.

   When I think about _____, I like _____
   and dislike _____ .
   When I think about _____, I like _____
   and dislike _____ .
   When I think about _____, I like _____
   and dislike _____ .

9. Begin practicing sharing your preferences with others. You will feel better as a result and you will help others learn to express their preferences.

   I will share my practices with others. _____yes
   After I've done this a few times, I realize that others _____
   _____ .

Your Commitments:

I commit to watch and listen to people's words and
   body language regarding their pleasure or discomfort
   with hugging and touching. _____yes

I will not press my preferences on anyone.   _____yes
I will be open about my preferences with others.   _____yes

What Makes This Hard To Do:

It's hard to realize that not everyone likes what you do. And it may also mean you won't always be able to get what you like. That's hard to give up.

It's also difficult to read another person if you expect the person to be a certain way and then he's not. An example of this would be a long-lost relative or an in-law whom you don't know well. You consider both *family*. But remember, just because they're family doesn't mean they like what you like or think the way you think.

GETTING COMFORTABLE WITH TOUCH

Question:

Do you find it hard to let your partner know what pleases you sexually?

Why This Happens:

- Each of us has different sensitivity to the amount and type of touch we prefer.
- The way in which the sensation of touch feels has nothing to do with how much we love a partner.
- You cannot tell by looking at someone what kind and how much touch the person likes and wants.
- There is generally a myth in this culture that makes couples think they ought to automatically know what each other likes and wants if they *love* one another.
- Words must convey the message. And in the beginning of an intimate relationship you must talk; otherwise, the displeasure will build into a giant block to intimacy if your feelings and preferences go unspoken.
- There is no right or wrong way of approaching lovemaking as long as both people desire the means.

Problems You Face Because You Get Uncomfortable with Touch:

- Even when you love your partner dearly, you find some physical activities stressful.
- Foreplay may get on your nerves.
- You feel trapped or weighted down by the other's closeness.
- You feel awful about how you feel.
- You hurt your partner's feelings without meaning to.
- Your partner doesn't understand your behavior and gets hurt.
- You shut down and close your partner out, damaging the relationship.

Your Goal:

Learn to communicate your preferences to your partner, clearly and without judgment.

What Not To Do:

Do not fail to communicate likes and dislikes about intimate touch.

Your Work:

1. Begin by telling the other person how much you love him or her and that you are excited about exploring how you can bring pleasure to him/her.
   I will have a heart-to-heart talk with my partner/friend at a time when the relationship is in a calm space. _____yes

2. Let inquisitiveness and curiosity be your guiding map. Don't assume you ought to know what to do or that there is one way of doing it.
   I will open my mind to many ways of achieving
      comfort with my partner.   _____yes
   I will remain open to the feelings of my partner.   _____yes
   I will make sure that judgment is not a part of
      our relationship.   _____yes

3. If you know you are sensitive to touch, tell your partner right away. Have this conversation when you are on sexually neutral ground, not when either of you is aroused or disappointed.
   You might say something like, "I've always been very sensitive to touch, honey. What feels good to most people usually doesn't feel good to me. I do like to be touched in some ways and can't stand to be touched in others. This has nothing to do with you, I promise. It's how I'm made."
   Ask your partner to work with you. If he or she is willing, share what you like and dislike. Demonstrate to your partner the pressure you like and the type of stroking.
   I would like to have this discussion with _____
   within the next _____ .
   I'd like to tell her/him the following: _____
   _____
   _____ .

4. If your partner has already unwittingly transgressed your comfort zone, doing something you don't like, tell him or her so, adding, "You didn't have any way of knowing."
   I will tell my partner _____
   that I don't like _____ .

Continue by saying, "I love that you want to please me." Then ask your partner to do something else to show the same affection—something with which you are comfortable.

I will tell my partner how much I love being touched by him/her and then will ask for something that feels comfortable, like _____

_____ .

5. More than likely, your lover will have a questioning look. Say how different kinds of touch feel to you. You may wish to mention how a little pressure may feel like a heavy weight on your shoulders. But then mention how to show the same affection with a little pressure.

I can do this. _____yes

6. Make "I" statements—that is, take responsibility for how you feel—instead of making "you" statements. "You press down too hard" puts the person off, while "I am very sensitive to any pressure" places the responsibility on you rather than on the other person.

I commit to making "I" statements and will restate what I said any time I forget and make a "you" statement. _____yes

7. Tell your partner "thank you" for being understanding. Then enjoy your mutually satisfying intimacy. You may have to guide your partner during lovemaking, but that is a natural part of bringing pleasure to another person. And have fun!

I will say "thank you" to my partner for understanding. _____yes

8. If your honey gets hurt feelings, just say, "This is my deal. It's only the way in which my brain and nerves are constructed. It's no reflection on you."

I can say this. _____yes

9. If your partner is critical of you or says "You *should* get over being so sensitive," say, "I'm as sensitive as I am. It's part of me. I hope you can understand and respect my wishes."

I will hold my own if I am criticized and told how I *should* be. _____yes

10. If your partner continues to criticize or shame you, consider getting out of the relationship quickly. Your desires and rights must be appreciated and honored. Besides, your partner is not available for a mutually pleasuring relationship.

After thinking about the relationship, I will decide if I want to leave the relationship. _____yes

I sense I'd like to _____ .

Your Commitments:

I commit to speak gently, truthfully, and with respect.   _____yes

I will make "I" statements, not accusing the other
   operson r placing responsibility on that person.   _____yes

I commit to do what is in the best interest of each
   nof us, ot one of us.   _____yes

What Makes This Hard To Do:

Most often it's the fear that you're not doing sex *right* that gets in the way, as you have an unrealistic expectation that true lovers and experienced sexual partners will automatically know what to do. There's also the fear that the other person won't continue to love you if you say anything. Actually, healthy true love can only grow with communication and sharing.

FEELING IN THE MOOD FOR SEX

Question:

Do you wonder why you have to "feel in the mood" for lovemaking while some people seem to be able to enjoy sex regardless of what their day has been like?

Why This Happens:

- Feelings-oriented people feel first rather than think about what is happening to them. If you're this way, you wear your feelings on your sleeve and are particularly susceptible to the effects of stress, hurt, and worry. You can't just *put your feeling aside.*
- Being sensitive to feelings means you will not be able to easily, if at all, override your feelings, especially when you're engaging in something like sex that also involves your feelings. Genuine intimate communication is heart-based. It touches your feelings deeply. So you must be "in the mood," if you're a feelings-oriented person.

Problems You Face Because of Your Need to Feel in the Mood for Sex:

- You and your partner get at odds about when to have sex.
- You feel guilty when you're not in the mood.
- Your partner doesn't think you love her/him, even though you do.

Your Goal:

To come to consensus solutions regarding your sexual relationship so both of you feel like winners.

What Not To Do:

Do not override your feelings because you think you *should*. Of course, don't wallow in them either.

Your Work:

1. Sensitively assess your needs and those of your mate, using your good thinking mind to decide whether to proceed at a given time or delay lovemaking between you.

> I commit to use my thinking mind instead of emy motions to decide whether to proceed at a given time with sex.   _____yes
>
> When I do think sex needs to be delayed, I will be honest and kind to my partner.   _____yes
>
> I will learn ways to work through this tough dilemma.   _____yes

2. Your sensitivity will very much affect your moods. Assess yourself during a neutral time when you're not making love. Ask yourself, "How sensitive am I to feelings and what happens to me when I'm stressed?" Do you take to heart what other people say or do? Does your mood shift, based on what's going on around you? Be sure to not judge your answers to these questions. But know that they will affect your mood.

   > Am I sensitive to feelings?   _____yes
   >
   > What happens to me when I'm stressed? _____
   >
   > _____
   >
   > Do I take to heart what other people say or do?   _____yes
   >
   > Does my mood shift, based on what's going on around me?   _____yes

3. Also, in a neutral time, talk with your spouse. Share what you've discovered about yourself. Then ask your spouse to consider the same questions with regard to himself or herself. Find out how your spouse is affected by stress and what gets him or her down. Discuss the similarities and differences without criticism or judgment.

   > I plan to share what I've learned about my sensitivity with _____ by (date) _____ .
   >
   > I will ask _____ how he/she is affected by stress.
   >
   > We came up with these similarities: _____
   >
   > _____
   >
   > _____ .
   >
   > We came up with these differences: _____
   >
   > _____
   >
   > _____ .

4. Devise a set of mental yardsticks to reflect what each of you desires. For example, you might use a scale numbered one to ten to measure the desire each of you has for sex. A one means "I don't want to have sex at all." Ten means "I'm dying to have sex." Let's suppose you rate yourself at a three and your spouse rates himself or herself at a seven. With

these scores, you have a tangible guide to help you both decide what to do at this moment.

I agree to use a mental yardstick to help my partner and me see
where we stand in relation to sex at a given time. _____yes

5. Clearly, without apology, compare your scale results with
   your partner's.

   When we compared our scale results, I rated myself with a
   _____ and my partner came up with a rating of _____.

6. When your partner is fairly eager for sexual relations and you
   are lukewarm, you need to decide whether you may be able
   to diffuse your stress after a little time or relaxing activities.
   For example, you might do some physical exercise, talk or
   journal through your feelings, meditate, have your partner
   give you a back rub, listen to music, read the newspaper, or
   sleep. Perhaps you'll be able to drain off the stressful feelings.
   Then you'll feel ready and eager to shift your attention to en-
   joying relations with your partner.

   I commit to try _____, _____, or
   _____ the next time I am not eager
   for sex and my partner is.

   The result of my doing _____ was _____
   _____ .

7. If you can't or don't want to get beyond your feelings at this
   time, say so. "I am not going to be able to get past my feelings right now." You might also say, "This is not a good time
   for me to enjoy sex. I'm sorry."

   I commit to tell the truth to my partner if I
      can't or don't want to get beyond my feelings.   _____yes
   I commit to say that it's my thing and not
      connected to my partner.
      (That's assuming it isn't.)   _____yes

8. Then, in the spirit of helping your partner get his or her needs
   met even though you don't want to have sex right then, ask
   what you can do for your partner. Make suggestions that you
   are willing to do. You might suggest getting together at a
   later time. Or if he or she is feeling very sexually aroused,
   volunteer to provide one-way pleasuring. This can be extremely satisfying to bring your partner pleasure without
   your being sexually aroused. Your pleasure comes from giving him or her pleasure.

This approach assumes your relationship is trusting and in pretty good shape. This is not to be used to override the tension in a marriage that is in trouble for other reasons and your sexual problems are the symptom of that trouble.

I am _____happy _____not willing to bring pleasure to my partner even when I'm not sexually in the mood.

This state of affairs is something that will only occasionally occur. If one of the partners continually is not in the mood for sex, that is a whole different issue and probably requires marriage and sex counseling.

9. If you absolutely do not want to engage in any stimulating involvement, say so and perhaps simply hold your partner tenderly. This lack of resolution can be a tender occurrence between you. Though lovers want to be there for each other, it simply is not always possible.

   Acknowledging the limits of your humanness can create a profound sharing, if it's done between two emotionally healthy individuals who understand their own and another's limitations. It can be a sweet time.

   I _____ have _____ have not known such moments of tenderness.

10. Under no circumstances make the result of your feelings your spouse's problem, such as by saying, "Why do *you* always want sex? *You* know I'm tired after work!" This puts the *blame* or responsibility onto him or her.

    I admit that I've placed blame.   _____yes
    I do not want to continue to do this.   _____yes
    I will work to change so I accept my l
       imitations and don't try to make someone
       else responsible for them.   _____yes

11. By the same token, do not let your spouse blame you for the way you are feeling and choosing to act as a result. Sexual relations are a mutually consenting enterprise, freely entered into by both partners.

    No blackmail, accusations, demands, or forced activities are acceptable. Shaming and blaming are not a part of a loving relationship. They are signs that an individual needs help with learning acceptable ways to get his or her needs met without hurting or trying to control another person.

I will not allow myself to be blamed for
   I am feeling and choosing to act.   _____yes
I will not be blackmailed.   _____yes
I am willing to seek counseling with my
   spouse to resolve these issues.   _____yes
I may even require it if I am to stay in the
   relationship.   _____yes

Your Commitments:

I commit to look openly and honestly at myself
   and my moods in relationship to my sex life.   _____yes
I commit to help my partner find fulfillment even
   if I'm not interested in sex at the time.   _____yes
I will not allow my partner to bully me into having
   sex if I do not desire to do so.   _____yes
I commit to seek counseling help if needed.   _____yes

What Makes This Hard To Do:

Many people come into intimate relationships without having learned how to communicate and resolve differences. There is also a lot of "illusion" and fantasy surrounding sex in our culture. It is not usually seen as a natural, mutually enjoyable, freedom-of-choice activity.

Fear plays a big role in individuals not caringly and gently speaking honestly about their needs. Fear of being left or disapproved of and feeling guilty are the most common. A healthy, loving relationship is never based on fear. Don't use it. Don't accept it.

FACING DENTISTS AND SHOTS

Question:

Do you abhor the thought of going to a dentist or getting a shot?

Why This Happens:

- Bodily sensitivity is determined by factors in your brain that are out of your control.
- Degrees of sensitivity vary greatly from one person to another. Pain generally is considered a subjective experience. However, people who are particularly sensitive to all stimuli may actually feel more pain than those who are less sensitive. You may be one of those people. If you are bothered by the tags in your clothing, imagine your reaction to shots and other bodily intrusions.
- Pain sensitivity doesn't change over time, though you can learn some techniques to help you get through the challenges.
- People who scold and blame others for their reactions either do not understand the differences between people or they are overcompensating because of their own discomfort. Overcompensation happens when someone doesn't face his or her own emotional reactions. Instead, he casts his feelings onto someone else, like you. If the person calls you a baby, in reality, he probably feels like a baby but is too ashamed to admit it.

Problems You Face When You Face Dentists and Shots:

- You experience fear.
- You avoid good health care because of your sensitivity.
- You feel ashamed at "being such a baby!"

Your Goal:

To eliminate the shame and self-deprecation you feel because of your sensitivity.

What Not To Do:

Do not accept the shame put on you or become self-critical.

Your Work:

1. Do protect your sensitive self and learn pain management techniques to make you more comfortable.
   I commit to protect myself.   _____yes
   I will learn pain management techniques.   _____yes
2. Immediately give yourself permission to be exactly as sensitive as you are. This means you are to stop thinking that you are somehow lacking because of your reactions.
   As hard as it is to believe that there's nothing inherently *wrong* with me because I'm sensitive, I will stop thinking that I am somehow lacking because of my reactions.   _____yes
3. Give yourself permission to be up front with others about how you are. Be matter-of-fact, saying, "I'm a sensitive person." With professionals, interview the person before committing yourself to his or her care. If the person brushes you off or doesn't acknowledge the importance of what you are saying, seek out someone else.

   Frequently, the professional is simply trying to stick to a schedule that doesn't allow the individualized attention you need. Some professionals are trained in techniques to assist with sensitive patients and clients. Others are not. Choose one who is empathetic and understands the issues at hand.
   I will review the professionals I know and only allow those who are willing to take the time to meet my individual needs to work with me. These include _____,
   _____, and _____ .
   When I meet with someone new, I'll share my
      need for assistance with my sensitivity and
      see how he or she reacts.   _____yes
   If I don't feel comfortable, I will see someone else. _____yes
4. Do not hesitate to ask for assistance from a professional to reduce or overcome your reaction to a procedure. Hypnosis and desensitization techniques can turn a scary or painful situation around to one that is quite tolerable. Medication may also be beneficial. Use whatever you are drawn to without feeling guilty or ashamed. Think of an anticipated visit to the dentist or for a procedure and visualize asking for assistance so you have a tolerable experience.
   I will ask for help with my next visit to the dentist or doctor.
   _____yes

5. Consider taking an advocate with you who understands you. Your advocate can assist you in getting what you want even if you're in the middle of a procedure. Your companion can also help you deal with your fears. Of course, you have to choose someone who knows what he or she is doing and doesn't feel embarrassed around authority or become nervous in such a situation.

   _____ or _____ would make good advocates for me to take.

   I will ask one of them to accompany me the next time I could use some support. _____yes

6. To family and friends who may have something negative to say about your sensitivity, simply set limits. "I prefer not to talk about it, and I sure don't want any criticism." This may seem harsh, but it's rude to disrespect another's needs and you don't deserve that treatment. You don't have to say it angrily, but in a matter-of-fact tone of voice. You can even give the person a hug as you say it.

   In my family, _____ often has something negative to say to me. I will speak directly to him/her and not accept the criticism any longer. _____yes

7. Learn self-hypnosis. Take a class or meet with a counselor who teaches this technique. It is simple and will do wonders to help you relax. You'll have a skill of value for life as a result.

   I will learn self-hypnosis in the following way: _____
   _____ .

   As a result, I now know what to do when I'm in a stressful situation. _____yes

   Dated _____ .

Your Commitments:

I commit to stand up for myself and my sensitivity.   _____yes

I will express my thankfulness and gratitude to those
   who help me.   _____yes

I see myself as strong and courageous as I accept
   help with my sensitivity.   _____yes

What Makes This Hard To Do:

Your own hesitation to stand up for yourself may cause you to suffer emotionally as well as physically.

RELIVING PAST PAIN

Question:

Does your mind replay hurtful events over and over?

Why This Happens:

- Traumatic experiences leave their mark on our emotions and intrude into our thought processes. As our minds struggle to deal with unacceptable, painful experiences, the whole ordeal may repeat itself in our minds. Parts of it cycle through our heads over and over and over again.
- Usually we think of traumatic events as such things as rape and sexual and physical assault, wartime experiences, or what happens to someone who is the victim of crime, an accident, or a severe illness. But everyday scoldings, criticisms, and humiliations have the same effect on sensitive, emotionally thin-skinned people. Even watching or hearing of these kinds of trauma-producing events or seeing them in movies or on TV can leave scars on those who are empathetic.
- Sensitive people are more likely to suffer traumatic reactions because of what is said to them. This is because more feeling gets through their defensive systems to traumatize them than they can handle. Folks who are able to let things roll off their backs or who look at things from an impersonal perspective suffer fewer traumatic reactions than people whose feelings act as their primary processing mode.
- Sometimes old memories of hurtful situations will trigger a reoccurrence of a past trauma. Let's say your boss criticizes you publicly. You may even feel and believe she is wrong, but you react nonetheless, as if you're being crucified. Long ago you may have suffered an incident that felt similar that you since *forgot* about until the current resurrection by your boss.
- In an active, creative mind, sometimes the fear of something happening simulates the actual happening of it, resulting in a trauma reaction.
- You are likely to experience a trauma reaction if you are brainwashed to believe that the True You is unacceptable or less than wonderful. Therefore, minority people as well as those who don't fit the cultural model of excellence are sub-

jected to trauma-producing beliefs. People whose brain construction is not linear experience this kind of assault to their self-esteem, which can be crippling to their sense of adequacy.

Problems You Face Because You Relive Your Past Pain:

- The Wounded You relives pain you experienced long ago.
- You feel confused and numb and may have trouble sleeping.
- You restrict your present life because of problems from your past.
- You just plain suffer.

Your Goal:

To take the steps needed to assist your psyche in truly healing from the trauma in your past.

What Not To Do:

Do not run away from the pain in any fashion or try to numb it with alcohol or drugs (prescription or street).

Your Work:

1. Immediately stop any wounding behavior that is being perpetrated on you now. You may say to any person committing an assault on you, physically or verbally, "That's enough." You can hold up your hand, palm facing toward the person speaking, or you can back off. Leave the room if necessary.
   I will immediately speak to _____
   who often verbally chastises me even though I'm grown up.
   I will no longer allow anyone to hurt me. I will stand up for myself or leave the situation immediately._____yes

2. Take a deep breath and begin to nurture yourself. You may immediately begin to rock, even while you're standing. You may visualize yourself hugging your vulnerable inner self. Maybe start to hum to yourself. Walk outside. Swing. Use whatever physical soothing feels good to you.
   I will self-nurture myself. _____yes
   I notice that I tend to _____
   _____ physically when I'm hurt.
   I will purposely do this behavior to soothe myself. _____yes

3. Call or go see someone you trust who will simply listen to you and offer support. You do not want someone to problem-solve at this stage. You most definitely do not want someone to tell you what you *should* or *could* have done differently.
I will seek out the help of _____
to listen to me and give me support.

4. If your personality is the type that tends to fight, you're likely to immediately criticize and verbally attack the person hurting you. You may put the person down. It's a cover-up for how badly hurt you feel. This is a natural response, though one that may get you in big trouble and eventually come around to hurt you. It also doesn't solve the true problem: healing the Wounded You.
I admit that I have the type of personality that
   tends to fight.   _____yes
I realize I need to come to grips with the hurt
   istored nside myself.   _____yes
I must remember that my true goal is to heal
   my Wounded Self.   _____yes

5. Check with yourself to see if you're ready to decide what you want to do about your healing. If you don't feel ready to do anything, don't do anything.
I _____am _____am not ready to decide what I want to do about my healing.

6. When you're ready to talk out the old wounding, consult a friend, cleric, or counselor. Journal the old experience and rewrite the old script so it has a different ending, one that is supportive, healing, and empowering.
I would like to talk to:
_____a friend, _____a cleric, _____a counselor, or _____other.
I would like to journal my old experiences and rewrite the script with a different ending. _____yes

7. When you're ready—remember, no rush—begin to look at your current situation objectively. Here are some guidelines in the form of questions to ask.
Was this a repetitive occurrence? _____yes
Does this person strike out only at me or all people?
_____only at me _____at everyone
Do the outbursts happen frequently or occasionally?
_____frequently _____occasionally
Have they only recently started to happen? _____yes _____no

8. When you have the answers to these questions, you will have a better idea of what you can and need to do about the abuse. The person may be under stress if the outbursts are recent. But regardless of what you learn, there is no reason for you to continue to be subjected to the abuse.
   Here's a summary of what I've gathered about the person and the abuse: _____
   _____ .

9. Next, decide if you want to have a discussion with the person. You can, or you don't have to. Depending upon the willingness or ability of the person to change, such a discussion may be useful.
   As I think about the person and the situation, I think the person _____may _____may not respond to a discussion.
   Either way, I _____will _____will not have a discussion with him or her.

10. Check the amount of all-around stress in your life. If you have a number of other sources of stress, you may wish to be extra protective of yourself. You may want to distance yourself more than if other parts of your life are stable.
    The level of stress in my life is _____low, _____medium, _____high.
    I need to distance myself from this situation. _____yes
    I am able, at this time, to deal with this situation. _____yes _____no

11. No job or relationship is worth being abused. You don't deserve it, though if you were an abuse victim since childhood, you may believe you do. That is for a counselor to help you heal.
    I _____do _____do not think or feel I deserve to be abused.
    I do not make the abuse happen. _____yes

12. There are always more jobs and more people with whom to create relationships.
    I need to consider alternatives to my present situation, on the job or personally. _____yes

13. Remember, you are your own advocate in the long run, even as you ask others to help you.
    I will serve as my own advocate. _____yes
    I deserve to protect and support myself. _____yes

14. Sometimes people do not mean to hurt you but do nonetheless. People who are not particularly sensitive to feelings can

walk over you with cleats and not know they're doing it. If the person isn't striking out because of having been wounded, you have a stronger likelihood of being able to remain in contact and educate him or her about your sensitivity. Then it would probably be safe to remain in a relationship.

I believe _____ does not mean to hurt me. I don't think he/she is not so wounded that striking out at me in order to feel better is necessary. _____yes

I am willing to remain in a relationship with him/her. _____yes

Your Commitments:

I commit to self-protect and self-support.   _____yes
I commit to no longer enable another to
   be an abuser using me or others as a victim.   _____yes
I commit to overcome the damage done to me
   as a child.   _____yes

What Makes This Hard To Do:

If you were abused or criticized as a child, you may not realize there is another way. Get counseling. You never deserved the abuse, and you now have a chance to break the cycle. You're worth it!

❺

Succeeding at Work

Throughout this book you've discovered the many ways in which brainstyle impacts how people deal with information and how they feel and behave. You've seen the uniqueness that each of us brings to society. You've watched how your talents and skills are shaped by the processing of your brain. You've learned many ways to utilize your uniqueness in the best interest of your True Self while learning to accommodate to environments that do not readily fit your natural ways, but in which you choose to function in order to achieve outcomes you desire.

The culmination of this understanding and skill building often expresses itself through your work. Whether you're dealing with short-term jobs or long-range career plans, the role played by your particular style of brain construction can give you an edge on success. It can also separate you from achieving your goals.

The True You automatically embraces the unique dreams that make up who you are. To the degree to which you recognize these dreams and follow your desires, you cannot help but succeed if you honor the natural way in which you are constructed. Yet everyday hindrances can act as blocks if you don't see them for what they are and know what to do about them. Ending up disappointed, saddened, and frustrated need not happen when you respect the way in which the True You works.

Through self-understanding and commitment to finding what fits you best on the job, your True Self will achieve the focus that will successfully lead you to your goals.

SUFFERING FROM FEELINGS OF INADEQUACY

Question:

Do you suffer from feelings of inadequacy about your work life?

Why This Happens:

- Different people hold different beliefs. Some people actually believe that one person or set of skills is superior to another. They will justify their beliefs by pointing toward education, amount of money made, social skills, and how serious a person takes life. Yet these are all culturally defined beliefs—they are judgments.
- If someone values "getting ahead" and keeping an orderly home or office, then that person may not realize that not everyone has these same priorities. Another person may value time spent with family and friends or in creative endeavors. Often a person leans in one direction or the other.
- Valuing tasks and skills shaped by a brainstyle different from your own will lead to feelings of inadequacy.
- To the degree you are trying to do work that doesn't naturally fit your brainstyle, no matter what that is, you will need to spend more time accomplishing the same task someone with a good fit to the work spends.
- If you are a hands-on, active, kinesthetic person trying to manage details and keep order, you are not likely to be drawing from your strengths. As a result, you'll be required to work very, very hard to just survive. You'll probably come up short even then. You are likely to feel like you're always catching up and never in control of what you're doing
- You may also feel inadequate if you are a creative visionary who has trouble translating your visions into reality. It's *so* easy for you to have the vision. It's *so* hard for you to manifest it. This is because you see the completed vision as perfect. But everyday life is not so perfect. Trying to perfectly replicate a dream at home or on the job can cause you to feel frustrated and let down. You still may not achieve a replica of your dream even with endless hours of trying—though you can achieve a satisfactory replica if you will allow yourself to be realistic and slightly less than perfect.

Problems You Face Because of Feeling Inadequate in Relation to Your Work:

- You are depressed or anxious a lot of the time.
- You feel that your talents and skills are not valuable.
- You feel you come up short in relation to your partner and other people.

Your Goal:

To learn the value of your innate gifts and their place in the scheme of things.

What Not To Do:

Do not assume that you have to work so hard all your life or constantly feel inadequate.

Your Work:

1. To figure out why you don't value yourself, you must assess why you work so hard. Then you can decide what to do about it.

   I work so hard because _____

   _____ .

2. Make two lists. On List 1, note what you like or even love about your jobs at home and in the workplace. Note what is easy for you to do. Note your strengths. Think of what you accomplish effortlessly on your job. You may not think of these strengths as valuable because they are so easy for you to do.

   List 1   List 2

   _____   _____
   _____   _____
   _____   _____
   _____   _____
   _____   _____
   _____   _____

3. Now figure out on List 2 how much of your time you currently spend doing what you don't like or what feels hard to do.

   I spend _____ percent of my time doing what I don't like to do or what feels hard to do.

4. If your natural attributes aren't being readily used, ask why you do what you do. Whose idea was it? Do you want to stay doing these things? How do you want to use your time?
Why am I doing what I am doing? _____

_____
Whose idea is it? _____
Do I want to continue to do these things? _____yes
I must be careful to do what I truly want to do, not what I *should* do. How do I want to use my time? _____

_____

5. You may have spent a lifetime being criticized, with one kind of accomplishment rated higher than another. Also, a lot of people haven't learned to put people first before accomplishments. Think about changing your mind-set.
How was I criticized and by whom? _____

_____
Was one kind of work or skill valued more than another?
_____yes
Which skills were valued highly? _____

_____
Did I have any of them? _____yes
Which of my skills were taken for granted? _____

_____

6. Recognize that there are different parts of you. There's the frightened part, which is the drudging, overworking part, and there's the part that does things easily. Now, remember the part of you that does things easily. Introduce that part to the frightened part of you. Tell the frightened part you appreciate how hard he or she has worked for you. Reassure the frightened part that he or she no longer has to attempt to do the things that are too hard. Thank the part that does things easily. As a result, you don't have to be so frightened.

Then take a breath and breathe in the new, hopeful attitude and breathe out the old, tense, frightened anger. Continue affirming the positive step with your in-breaths and exhale the old, bad feelings and tension with the out-breaths.
I am willing to do this exercise. _____yes

7. Become clear about what you have to offer.

I have _____

_____ to offer.

8. If you're a creative visionary with a desire to replicate your dreams in everyday life, you will need to be aware that this is what you're doing. If you let the perfect representation of your desire rule your actions, you can work yourself into a frenzy. If you take the time to think through your situation and what you want to do about it, however, you can get in the driver's seat, making choices that are in your best interest. To do this, consider the audience or recipient of your creative work. Ask the following questions:

How appreciative are they of my finished product? _____

_____

What is the use to which my work is to be put? _____

_____

Do I want or need to put in the
   amount of time it will take to
   create near perfect work?   _____yes _____no
Do I have a better use for my time?   _____yes _____no
Are there other projects that are
   getting bumped, maybe never to
   be done, because I'm spending so
   much time on this one?   _____yes _____no

9. Once you've answered these questions, you can make a conscious choice about how you want to spend your time. You can work from your strengths and clearly decide how much time you want to spend manifesting your visions.

I choose to work from my strengths. _____yes

If you checked "yes," then continue.

I choose _____

_____

_____.

10. As a visionary, you must also realize that it takes time for the implementation of your visions to become functional in daily life. Patience is called for.

I realize I am a visionary.   _____yes
I realize it takes time for the implementation
   of my visions in daily life.   _____yes
I will be patient.   _____yes

Your Commitments:

I commit to make the choices that I desire to make.   _____yes
I commit to be honest with myself and take
   responsibility for who I am.   _____yes
I no longer am willing to feel inadequate.   _____yes

What Makes This Hard To Do:

Many people think there's status in working exceedingly hard. It's a cultural belief that it is saintly to give 110 percent all the time. It's not. It's not even possible.

Another attraction to working so hard is that others admire your tenacity without realizing all that work may not be benefiting you or anyone else. You'll need to give up outside approval, face a reevaluation of how you spend your time, and be sure you're living by your own inner beliefs, not those of someone else.

TAKING TESTS

Question:

Does test taking feel nightmarish to you?

Why This Happens:

- The types of tests all of us prefer to take, whether at work or school, are those on which we can do well—that is, ones that most accurately measure what we know and allow us to show what we know.
- The types of tests on which we do best are a reflection of our style of brain construction.
- To the degree to which you are a person who sees the big picture and recalls the function of something rather than its name, you will do poorly on fill-in-the-blank and multiple-choice questions. If you learn and work kinesthetically, you will prefer demonstrations or open-ended, descriptive tests to those requiring you to recall details and labels.
- Answers to multiple-choice tests often have slight variations in their content—variations that big-picture people have trouble seeing. You are likely to become confused when you're trying to compare details. You know the difference when you're doing your job, but reading about it, out of context, doesn't reflect what you know. If you could write a description of how to do your job, you would probably show clearly the subtleties that you miss on a multiple-choice test.

Problems You Face When You Take Tests:

- You may be unable to show what you know or can do in real life by taking a test.
- You feel anxious and don't do well even when you try.
- You fall behind at work because you can't get good grades on job-related tests.

Your Goal:

To demonstrate on tests what you know or to be evaluated in a way that is fair.

What Not To Do:

Do not give up seeking job advancement or an education.

Your Work:

1. You must learn to beat the tests or get around them. Either way works in your behalf.

   Because of my brainstyle, I may have to work harder on certain kinds of tests. I am willing to do this if I'm able. _____yes

   Sometimes, though, no matter how hard I try, I can't show what I know on a test. Then I must find an alternative way to get to my goal. _____yes

2. On the job or in school, you can request that a test of the knowledge needed for your new job be given in a form that shows what you know. Through the Americans with Disabilities Act, you have the legal right to be tested in a form that fits your particular style of brain construction. You can ask that the test be given orally or that you demonstrate what you know. (See "Returning to College" in chapter 2; for ADA guidelines, see the section below and the addendum, "The Americans with Disabilities Act," for additional job-related comments.)

   I will become familiar with the options that are available through the Americans with Disabilities Act. Using it doesn't mean there is something *wrong* with me, however. _____yes

3. On the job you may not need to go as far as formally instigating ADA. Instead, you can ask your current supervisor at work to informally request a dispensation from the formal test. Or the boss or someone who is your supporter may be willing to write a letter of support for you and explain your situation.

   I will ask my supervisor or boss to either grant me a dispensation from formal testing or write a letter on my behalf to support me in the job situation. _____yes

4. If you are required to proceed with the testing in its original form, study with someone in the company who is familiar with the test. Go over and over tests like the one you'll be taking. Have your tutor point out the subtle differences between answers so you can learn to think like the person scoring the test.

I think _____ would make a good tutor for me to study with. I will contact him/her and lay out a study plan.

5. Make a suggestion to those people in the company who are responsible for advancement as well as hiring procedure to become familiar with brain diversity and the assessment needs of various individuals.

    I will advocate for personnel service employees
       and managers to become familiar with
       differences in brainstyle and how it affects
       test taking.   _____yes

    I will talk to our employee groups about
       brainstyles.   _____yes

    I will arrange a speaker to come to the employee
       group's or manager's meeting to talk about
       brainstyles and testing.   _____yes

6. If you are in training or school, get to know your professor's testing preferences. Even before you register for a class, talk with the person. Also ask other students, special needs counselors, and student-friendly professors which professors will fit your learning style best. If at all possible, only take classes from those professors who give tests that your brainstyle allows you to handle successfully to demonstrate what you know.

    I agree to seek out teachers before I register for classes. _____yes
    The following professors/teachers test in ways that I can show what I know:

_____

_____ .

7. In school, tell your professor about your difficulty taking tests. Ask if you can show her or him in others ways that you can do the work. Ask for extra credit.

    I am willing to do all I can do to pass my classes.   _____yes
    I will ask for alternative testing.   _____yes
    I will ask for extra credit.   _____yes

Your Commitments:

I commit to responsibly prepare for testing.   _____yes
I also will speak up about the types of testing
    that will best show what I can do.   _____yes

I will advocate for myself and others so that
    I am/we are fairly treated with regard to job
    advancement and the mastery of class material.   _____yes
If necessary, I will use the Americans with
    Disabilities Act to open a legal door to give me
    a fair chance in the workplace and in school.   _____yes

What Makes This Hard To Do:

Many people hold an untrue assumption that if you know the material being tested you will do well on any test. Others simply don't understand that there is a difference between types of tests and not everyone does equally well on all kinds. You must become wise about tests and pass on your wisdom to others.

Addendum: The Americans with Disabilities Act

1. Everything mentioned in the section entitled "Returning to College" also applies in the workplace. For example, if you are a salesperson and do that job well, you can ask for help with your clerical work. You can ask for flextime so you can come in early or stay late to do your paperwork when the office is quiet.
2. On the job you generally do not need to make a big deal of *demanding* accommodation. You don't even need to say that you have a special need supported by testing. Simply provide your employer with information about how you can do your job best. Many will accommodate you to that end.
3. Of course, if you feel blocked from doing a good job, if your reasonable requests are turned down, or if you are poorly rated because of an unaccommodated need, you may wish to use the ADA to get what you need to do a quality job.

ASSESSING JOB-HOPPING

Question:

Does your resume have lots of jobs listed, many of which you stayed in for only a short period?

Why This Happens:

- Sometimes job changes are in your best interest and sometimes they are not. If you're starting on a career track where one job leads to another and another, you may be moving each time you quickly master a step. You may find you're moving upward with increases in pay, status, and responsibility.
- This will tend to happen when you're in a growing field and you have a visionary picture of where you want to go. This means, of course, that you are a big-picture kind of person. You probably have a dream, one that both motivates you and urges you on toward completion.
- If you're a bright, creative person who tires quickly in any job you master, you will more than likely move on to a job from which you can learn. However, it is also possible that the pain of remaining static is so great that you quit before you have something else.
- You may get easily bored in jobs with a lot of repetition or where there's little chance for creativity or ingenuity. As a result, you feel stressed and *have* to move. This tends to happen when you have the kind of brain that likes stimulation and can process information and experiences quickly. Again, you may move responsibly or without thought depending upon the amount of training you've had to accommodate the way in which your brain is constructed. (See "Escaping Boredom" in the next section.)
- Of course, it's always possible that you have to move on because you can't get along with people, have authority issues (see "Displacing Your Anger onto Others" in chapter 3), have an issue with addiction, or are unable to handle the job responsibly.

Problems You Face Because of Job-Hopping:

- You may create a poor-looking resume.
- Others consider you unstable.

- You worry that you won't be able to progress in the work world.
- You worry you aren't mature.

Your Goal:

Assess carefully and honestly the reasons you change jobs.

What Not To Do:

Do not automatically assume there is something wrong with you because you don't stick with a job for a long period of time.

Your Work:

1. Look carefully at the reasons you change jobs. Are you moving because it is in your best interest?
   I open my mind to the reasons behind my
      job changes.   _____yes
   I consider whether my moves are wise or
      symptomatic of problems in me.   _____yes

2. Begin to sort through the changes you've made job-wise by listing the jobs you've had in the last several years and the reasons you've left. You can do this on paper, in your mind, or talking to someone else. You must be absolutely honest with yourself.

   Jobs I've left   The reasons I left

   _____   _____
   _____   _____
   _____   _____
   _____   _____
   _____   _____
   _____   _____
   _____   _____

   If you run out of room, continue on a lined sheet of paper.

3. Check to see if you have a big picture in your mind, one that reflects where you're headed career-wise. Ask yourself if you have a dream or a vision you'd like to fulfill. Is that what drives you?
   Do I have a big picture in my mind—one that will affect me career-wise? _____yes _____no
   Here's a description of my picture:_____

_____
_____.

Do I have a dream or a vision I'd like to fulfill?

_____yes _____no

I am driven by _____a picture, _____a dream, _____a vision.

Here's what my dream or vision looks like: _____

_____.

4. Now check to see which of your job moves has brought you closer to the completion of your goal. If each has, you can relax about the changes you've made.

When I look at the job moves I've made and dreams, pictures, and visions I hold in my head, they seem to fit together.

_____yes _____no

5. Every single change may not have turned out to be to your benefit. That does not necessarily mean you have a problem. Ask yourself what you learned from any ill-fated change. Do you sense you made a mistake? What did you learn from that error, and how are you using that information now?

I can think of _____ changes that did not benefit me directly. They are _____

_____.

Look again at potential benefits that may have accrued, perhaps not directly, but that eventually helped you or are helping you reach your goal.

When I look again, I see the benefit of these moves. _____

_____.

What have I learned from any ill-fated changes? _____

_____
_____.

Do I sense I made a mistake? _____yes, _____not necessarily, _____no

What have I learned from my errors? _____

_____
_____.

I am now using that information in the following ways: _____

_____
_____.

6. Note whether you've made the same mistake several times. That's a sign you need help with a pattern that's not in your best interest. Be brutally honest with yourself. What do you

need to fix in yourself? You may need to seek consultation or counseling to get past this speed bump in your path.

I have made the same mistake several times. It is _____
_____ .

What do I need to fix it? _____
_____ .

I am willing to seek counseling to help me get past this problem. _____yes _____no

If your answer is "no" then what are you willing to do?

I am willing to _____
_____ .

7. If you get bored with jobs, you are either underemployed, doing a job with lower expectations than you are capable of meeting, need more education so you can get a more challenging job, or are in the wrong kind of job.

I get bored with my jobs because _____
_____ .

8. If you get easily bored, consider a job where the assignment continually changes. Some likely candidates include jobs with troubleshooting assignments or creative design (in any field), or a job with regular new assignments such as patent law, counseling, or custom building.

Since I do get bored easily, I will think of jobs that change in and of themselves, such _____
_____ .

9. If you are underemployed, you either need to go back to school, get additional training, or invent a new job that requires you to learn a lot on your own. For example, if you've been a physician's assistant but keep job-hopping because you get tired of the work, you may need to become a physician so you are freed of the limitations your training has If you've been in the building trades but are tired of going from job to job where you do the same thing over and over, you may want to start your own business or design a building product for which you handle the marketing placed on you.

I would like to _____
_____
_____ .

10. If you job-hop because you can't do the job, you need to look at your initial choice of jobs and seek one that fits you better. I would feel relief being out of the kind of job I've been doing. What I'd really like to do is _____
_____.

11. If you job-hop because you lose your temper, have a chemical dependency problem, or can't get along with people, you need counseling to get your emotions and your behavior under control. You deserve to do this for yourself.
When I look honestly at myself, I can see that my problem is _____
_____.
I agree I need counseling. _____yes _____no
If I don't want counseling, I will instead solve my problems by _____
_____.

Your Commitments:

I commit to appreciate the opportunities to move quickly from job to job toward my dreams.	_____yes
I commit to make the educational and training changes I need to improve my interest in my job.	_____yes
I commit to try out something totally new so that I can live up to my potential.	_____yes
I commit to get help with my chemical dependency or behavior or emotional problems.	_____yes

What Makes This Hard To Do:

The hardest part of remedying job-hopping is being honest with yourself about the reason(s) for changes. Be sure that what you're doing is truly in your best interest.

ESCAPING BOREDOM

Question:

Is boredom one of the greatest fears you face?

Why This Happens:

- When you have a quick-processing, big-picture mind, you rapidly understand what's happening. You may not need to hear all the words in a sentence or see all the steps of something to know the outcome. Unlike people whose brains are constructed in a detail-oriented, step-by-step way, people who require all the details before the big picture comes together for them, you see whole patterns immediately.
- You love the feeling of newness. It makes you feel good, almost high. It brings great zest to your life. There's nothing wrong with this, though those who don't understand sometimes think of newness as an addiction. It's only an addiction if it controls your life in a way that causes you trouble or is used to cover feelings with which you don't want to deal. A healthy love of new challenges can provide you with an interesting life with quality advancement.
- Boredom is an indicator that you're doing something that doesn't fit you.
- It can mean you're wasting time. That saps your life energy and shuts you off from experience, which feels bad when you're a lively, creative, curious person.

Problems You Face Because of Boredom:

- You feel bad, depressed, and angry and you feel like quitting what you're doing.
- You get restless and want to keep on the move, even when it means not doing the responsible thing.

Your Goal:

To pay attention to the messages and function of boredom and steer your life's course accordingly.

What Not To Do:

Do not try to force yourself to ignore your feelings of boredom.

Your Work:

1. Review your feelings of boredom from previous years. Ask yourself under what circumstances they occurred. What were you doing or not doing?
   Here's what I was doing or not doing when I was bored in the past: _____
   _____ .

2. Review the times in your life, including the present time, when you felt zestful and boredom-free. What were you doing? You'll learn a lot about your needs and life path by tackling these questions.
   When I felt zestful and boredom-free, I was _____
   _____
   _____ .

3. Ask yourself if you have a dream. Ask if you get bored when you're not following it or some other special interest.
   When I'm not following my dream or a special interest, I feel
   _____
   _____ .

4. Ask whether you use activity and change to soothe feelings of boredom. When you feel good as a result, do you make constructive use of that energy, propelling yourself toward a goal of your choosing or toward your dream? Or do you use the high to escape from dealing with feelings or situations that need attention?
   The answers to these questions will tell you whether you have an addiction to change or can use signs of boredom creatively as a guide for constructive living.
   How do I use activity and change? _____
   _____ .

   Do I use them to soothe my feelings
   of boredom?   _____yes _____no
   When I feel good as a result of activity
   and change, do I use the energy to
   move toward my dream?   _____yes _____no
   Do I use the energy to escape from
   wdealing ith my feelings or situations
   that need attention?   _____yes _____no
   I think I use activity and change in a
   constructive way.   _____yes
   I worry that maybe I have an addiction
   to change and activity.   _____yes

5. When others fear you're being irresponsible because you make changes when you're bored, check within yourself and consider the work you've done. Then you'll know whether to ignore their concern or take it to heart.

   If you honestly feel the accusation doesn't fit, tell the person, "Thank you for your concern. I'll take responsibility for any changes I make." Of course, you must then follow through responsibly.

   I am willing to take responsibility even
   though some people in my family or my
   friends are concerned that I use change
   inappropriately.   _____yes
   I will tell them that I will take care of
   the situation.   _____yes

6. Check to see how you handle situations in which you become bored. Ask yourself the follow questions:

   Do I bolt, leaving a mess of unfinished
   business behind me?   _____yes
   Do I face my commitments and responsibly
   take steps to extricate myself, such as giving
   notice on the job rather than walking out?   _____yes
   Do I have a dream, plan, or goal in mind that
   I want to follow?   _____yes
   Can I use feelings of boredom to determine
   whether I'm on the path to my dreams and
   goals or have gotten off my path?   _____yes

7. Use boredom constructively to guide you to the style of life that fits you, while acting respectfully to those around you.

   I will do this. _____yes

Your Commitments:

I commit to be truthful about my use of change
   in my life.   _____yes
I commit to follow the message of boredom in
   search of
   fulfillment of my dreams.   _____yes

What Makes This Hard To Do:

If you think you *should* remain in certain situations even though they bore you, you will struggle, unable to live authentically in relation to your True Self.

FINDING JOBS THAT FIT

Question:

Do you know what kind of job fits you?

Why This Happens:

- You must realize that not all people, no mater what their brainstyle, have similar interests, skills, and personalities.
- As a direct salesperson, you may be in a job that makes excellent use of your brainstyle and personality. After all, that's why you are good at what you do. You are in a right fit for someone who needs a high level of physical activity. Your ability to do more than one thing at a time and to express the naturally outgoing person you are is an asset.
- Others often inadvertently make suggestions to you that fit them without realizing that all people aren't made the same way. If you are not drawn to technical things, that's a sure sign that technical things aren't compatible with the way you are made. It doesn't matter how much money someone, somewhere is making or how many predictions say a particular job is the way the marketplace is going. If you don't like it, you'll feel miserable trying to do it.

Problems You Face Finding a Job That Fits:

- You become frustrated trying to use traditional ways to seek employment.
- You can find a job, but not one that you like.
- You become anxious, scared, depressed, and frustrated trying to fit into the workplace.
- You wonder if you *should* try to fit in so you can be responsible.

Your Goal:

To find a job that fits you and that you like, while still being a productive, responsible wage earner and citizen.

What Not To Do:

Do not try to do what someone else does just because the person thinks their way is *the* way.

Your Work:

1. Begin by scrutinizing your feelings and interests, noting what attracts and repels you.
   I have these interests: _____
   _____ .
   I do not like _____
   _____ .

2. Be sure to look at careers that not only take your style of brain construction into account but that also support your temperament, personality, and interests.
   When I consider jobs and careers I will factor in all sides of myself. _____yes

3. Then do not discuss your quest with anyone who isn't able to look at options through your eyes rather than their own. This is a skill that only some people have developed. It's precious. Only share with those who leave you feeling enthusiastic, positive, and hopeful about yourself and your future.
   I will share my quest with _____
   _____ .
   I will not share it with _____
   _____ .

4. Thank anyone who makes suggestions to you, and tell them you are carefully studying your options.
   I will do this. _____yes

5. Give yourself permission to follow a career track that you love, one that excites you and allows you to be who you are.
   I give myself permission to follow a career track that I love— one that excites me and allows me to be who I am. _____yes

6. Take an inventory of times and situations in your life when you were happy. Ask yourself what you were doing.
   When I was really happy, I was _____
   _____
   _____ .

7. Take a similar inventory of times and situations when you were unhappy, bored, or frustrated. Notice when your performance was lackluster and you resisted getting out of bed in the morning.
   When I was really unhappy, bored, or frustrated, I was _____
   _____
   _____ .

8. Get to know yourself well. Spend time reviewing your life. As I mull over my feelings in relation to past jobs or careers, I find that I _____

_____ .

9. If you're offered a job change or promotion, look carefully at the requirements of the new setting to find out if they fit you. Often, promotions in a company can mean a change from something that fits you to something that is a complete misfit. Preferably try out the change before you commit to the job. This is like trying on a suit of clothes before buying it. If this is not possible, ask lots of questions about what you'll actually be doing, how you'll be doing it, and how you'll be evaluated.
   I can see myself checking out a promotion or any job options this way. _____yes

10. Do not be blinded by offers of increased status and money. Though tempting, you must stay true to yourself and what you feel is important.
    I can see myself going beyond status and
       money to a job situation that I love.   _____yes
    I cannot see myself turning down status
       or money for a job I would love.   _____yes
    The reason I couldn't turn down the status is _____

    _____ .

    The reason I couldn't turn down the money is _____

    _____ .

11. Think of yourself. Though the person offering you the position may have been around longer and has more status than you, you know more about yourself, your innate strengths, weaknesses, and preferences as they are dictated by your brain construction. You must take responsibility in this area. When I think of _____, who has more experience than I do, I realize that I know more about myself than he/she does. _____yes

12. If you get in a job that ends up not being a good fit for you, don't wait for things to crumble around you. Immediately go to your boss and ask for help solving the situation. Be willing to leave the job in good graces. There's no disgrace in owning up to being a poor match for a particular situation. You will be admired for your keen observation and honesty.

I feel _____ about owning up to taking
the wrong job.

I believe I can overcome any fear that I feel, however. _____yes
I will step forward and take responsibility to get out of the
situation rather than being forced out or simply allowing
my job to disintegrate around me. _____yes

13. Take your values and courage in your hands and do the kind
of work that fits you. Life will continue with ups and down,
whether you're doing something you like or something you
dislike. You might as well do what fits you.

I commit to seeking a job that fits me.   _____yes

I am not at a place where I will allow myself
    to seek what fits me.   _____yes

I will consider working toward finding my fit
    in the future.   _____yes

14. Find or create a personal cheering squad that knows and values you as a person the way you are.

I cheer for myself. _____yes

I ask _____, _____,
and _____ to join me on my cheering squad.

Your Commitments:

I commit to work in ways that fit me.   _____yes

I commit to find jobs or a career that I like,
    even love.   _____yes

I will protect myself from undue outside influence
    to do something that doesn't feel right to me.   _____yes

What Makes This Hard To Do:

You will need to remain strong within yourself. Many people will
fail to understand what you're doing and why you're doing it. Surround yourself with supporters who believe in your ability to find
your own answers.

IMPLEMENTING YOUR DREAM

Question:

Do you fear you'll not be able to reach your dream job?

Why This Happens:

- For people with a creative, kinesthetic, visionary style of brain construction, the skills required to get through school are usually quite different from those upon which success after school depends. So you may be creatively brilliant, a great leader, a superb producer/networker, inventor, or troubleshooter/fixer, but have bland grades from your formal studies. You probably also have learned a lot outside of school on your own and through experience.
- You've not realized any of your dreams and don't even know where to begin. But you must realize that focusing on your talents and then finding ways to implement them takes time, experience, know-how, and courage.
- Finding and deciding which talents you want to make use of to reach your goal is a big job. They can be specific such as musical or artistic. They may be in the area of fixing or designing things or making friends. They can also be more complex, using multiple smaller skills. You may have the ability to problem-solve, be inventive, entrepreneurial, or able to network with people, bringing them together for teamwork. Your talent(s) may be in reading other people or managing details, being empathetic or psychic, leading others, or being a caregiver.
- Talent-based skills do not necessarily show up when you are young, especially if you do okay in school. You may not find them until later in your life. The more complex the talent or set of talents you possess, the longer it may take you to find them and use them.
- If you tend to be a big-picture person who likes variability and multitasking, you may become quite frustrated with traditional job roles. You may also job-hop, failing to stick to one thing for very long. Even so, you could be heading to your dream even if you don't realize that's what you're doing. You must ultimately realize you can put together the experiences you absorb from each job.

- If you have a sense, however, of "specialness," but are also frustrated, you probably haven't yet synthesized the elements that must come together for you on your life pathway. Remember, though, you wouldn't feel special if you weren't.
- Finding your dream path is only step one. There are many steps involved in implementing it and there are many ways to take those steps. There is always a path that fits the way your brain is constructed. Living your dream is a process that can take the rest of your life. You can't know all the steps at first because many will unfold only as you move forward and increasingly see new options from which to choose.
- Any time you get physical reactions to plans you've made so that you feel bad, know you're trying to do something in a way that isn't right for you. Similarly, if you have a negative reaction to a suggestion about how to proceed, it may be the wrong path for you to follow.
- Also, if you're trying to implement a dream—a dream that you arrived at through your feelings—you must manifest the dream by using your feelings. To switch to trying to implement it with strategic, linear thinking means you are scrambling for approval. Keep your feelings in the leadership role. Be consistent with the process that works for you.

Problems You Face Implementing Your Dream Job:

- Fear of overrating yourself.
- Fear of criticism from others.
- Depression at the thought of not being able to implement it.
- Not knowing how to go about implementing it.
- Fear of wasting your time trying.

Your Goal:

To become all that you ever dreamed of becoming by synthesizing your talents, interests, and desire.

What Not To Do:

Do not discount your feeling of specialness or let anyone tell you that you ought not to try to live out your heart's feelings.

Your Work:

1. Begin by giving yourself time to be introspective.
   I will set time aside to be introspective. Here are times when
   I can do this: _____ .

2. Keep a journal or somehow record your day and night dreams
   and your visions. Include dialogue. Note interests to which
   you are drawn and those experiences that turn you off.
   Day dreams: _____
   _____
   _____ .

   Night dreams: _____
   _____
   _____ .

   Interests to which I am drawn: _____
   _____
   _____ .

   Experiences that turn me off: _____
   _____
   _____ .

3. Review what you've done without judging it. For example,
   let's say you were involved in a venture that got you into
   trouble. Rather than discounting the whole experience as one
   big mistake to be wiped off your life-experience slate, review
   what you liked about it. Note what you hoped for and what
   excited you.
   I commit to not judge what happened, but rather look at what
   went wrong, what I liked, and what excited me. _____yes
   What excited me was _____
   _____

4. Next, pay attention to what went wrong. Ask yourself these
   questions:
   What was I hoping for that didn't work? _____
   _____ .

   Did I try to go too fast or want too much
      too soon?   _____yes _____no
   Was I trying to skim corners or did I fail to
      be totally honest?   _____yes _____no
   Did I stop believing in myself?   _____yes _____no
   Did I run into obstacles I didn't know how
      to solve?   _____yes _____no

Did I run out of money?   _____yes _____no
Did I trust people who turned out to
     be unreliable?   _____yes _____no

5. Look for patterns in what worked for and against you.
   I see a pattern that worked _____for _____against me. It
   looked like this: _____
   _____.

6. Search for people whose lives you admire. Ask why you ad-
   mire them.
   I admire _____, _____,
   _____, and _____.
   Why do I admire them? _____
   _____.
   What did they do that I like? _____.

7. Notice what you cannot keep yourself from doing. You'll repeatedly go back to activities or interests that are right for
   you. Be careful not to judge yourself at this time, leaving out
   activities or things that you feel or have been told are "foolish," "childish," or should be relegated to the category
   called "hobby."
   Reconsidering things that may have been labeled as "foolish,"
   "childish," or "hobby-material," I will add _____
   _____.

8. Now let your mind and heart soar. Just suppose that you actually can become anything you want to become. Let go!
   When I let myself go, I think of _____
   _____.

9. Once you've arrived at a dream choice or choices, all you
   have to do for now is take one step. That first step may be
   simple or complex. If the first step is clear, then just take it.
   My first step is _____clear _____complex.
   If it's clear I can take it now. It is _____
   _____.

10. If your task is complex, you will need to spend time looking
    at a number of ways you might proceed. Your job now is to
    decide which pathway will lead you to your goal.
    My task is complex, so I now realize I will need to look at a
    number of ways to proceed. _____yes

11. In deciding which path to use to proceed toward your goals,
    again listen to the feelings within yourself. Watch your re-
    action to suggestions from others or even to the so-called
    sensible voices from within. Let yourself meditate, and then

ask, "What's my next step?" (See the next section, "Creating in Your Mind.")

First, I will listen to my feelings in everything
   I do and am exposed to in the next while.   _____yes
I will become aware of "sensible" voices from
   within myself and see how I feel about them.   _____yes
If I feel uptight, I'll say "thank you" to the
   voice and then release it. If what I hear
   sounds good, I'll embrace what I hear and
   act on it and also say, "thank you."   _____yes
I will also meditate and then ask, "What's my
   next step," followed with being very observant. _____yes

12. Ask, "How can I find my next steps?" Watch and listen for an answer to your question. Note who calls or crosses your path. Pay attention to any interest that you start thinking about. Even notice if you are drawn to a book, including fiction, or a play, or a weekend activity. Though what you're attracted to may not make sense on the surface, it'll fit perfectly into your total plan.

    If you are trying this approach right now, list some of the things you are attracted to. _____
    _____

13. Ask, "How can I get the skills that I will need to proceed?" Look around for people you know who have them. The people don't necessarily need to be close to you.

    When I look around, I see people with skills I want to develop. These people are: _____
    _____ .

14. If schooling is involved, look at various ways to get that training. If credentials are needed and you feel overwhelmed about getting them or simply don't want to, do one of two things. Look for a way to practice your dream in a nontraditional way. Avoid steps that are particularly repugnant to you or, alternately, see if you can acquire the training and subsequent credential in a way that you can manage. (See "Returning to College" in chapter 2.)

    I _____ do _____ do not want to go back to school.
    If you don't want to return school, how can you practice your dream in a nontraditional way?
    I can think of several alternatives. _____
    _____
    _____ .

I also may be able to acquire training and credentials in the following way:

_____

_____

_____ .

15. For example, if you want to help people who are elderly but the idea of getting a degree in gerontology or counseling or social work worries you, look at alternative ways to reach your goal. You might start your own business. As a businessperson, you don't need a degree. You might go into partnership with someone who has the required degree or certificates so you can do what you do well and that person meets the legal requirements.
Thinking about alternative ways to do what I want, I can think of _____

_____ .
If I were to go into a business in the field in which I'm interested, I could start a _____ business.
I can even think of someone I might like to partner with.

_____

_____ .

16. Or, on a different track, you might host a television or radio show about and for older people. You could create plays and tour to places where older people live, putting on shows. You might include retirement home residents in the plays. You could lead elders on tours or design interiors or clothing or sport's equipment for older people. How about fundraising or ministering to the elderly? Your choices of ways to work with the elderly are endless.
As I extend my thinking about the area I'd like to work in I can brainstorm, coming up with many ideas. Some of them are _____

_____

_____ .

17. If you cringe at the thought of doing a business plan, don't do it. If the idea of a budget overwhelms you, set it aside for now. Later, when money becomes an issue for you to grow, you will notice the right person to help you learn what to do. Or you'll find a partner to take over the job. Or you'll be ready to face the budget yourself.
I feel _____ at the idea that I don't have to do a business plan.

I feel _____ that I can set budget issues aside for now. Later I can partner with someone to help with these issues or hire them out. I have choices and that feels

_____

18. Ask yourself if you dare put your dreams out into the world to become a reality. If you can't, ask why.
Whose voice do I hear in my mind, saying, "Oh, come on! Who do you think _____ .
From where are the limitations coming that I am bumping into? _____

_____

These limitations were learned, you know.
19. Realize that subsequent steps to making your dream a reality may take time. Make that time enjoyable. Learn a lot, try a lot, and be sure to affirm the way in which you work, honoring your styles of creation and implementation. Be flexible.
I agree that it may take time to live my dream.   _____yes
I will make that time enjoyable.   _____yes
I will be flexible in how I get to my dream.   _____yes
20. Don't stop unless you truly have a change of heart, but do take breaks.
I will work toward the goal to which
   I'm committed.   _____yes
If I have a change of heart, I will let myself
   release the goal and stop working toward it.   _____yes
I will take breaks.   _____yes

Your Commitments:

I commit to pursue my dreams as long as I desire
   to do so.   _____yes
I will find alternative routes when I bump into
   obstacles.   _____yes
I commit to be my own best ally.   _____yes

What Makes This Hard To Do:

Too often we are taught that dreams belong to childhood or there is a standard way of doing things. We give up our dreams figuring that they are foolish. Or we forfeit our dreams because the way we were trying to achieve them didn't work. Instead, brush off a dream, go back to the drawing board, and try another pathway toward the fulfillment to it. Resist being seduced by the approval of others.

CREATING IN YOUR MIND

Question:

Do you often have creative insights, thoughts, and solutions in your mind without planning to?

Why This Happens:

- The True You is a big-picture person who can draw from an infinite resource of potential bits of information within your brain. Your strength is in the relationships and processes between things. So your mind naturally tries out various details in different combinations and instantly recognizes those that please you or fit a situation. You can count on this process to fit the form or outline of an assignment even though you don't purposely *think* about it.
- You are capable of multitasking. You can think of more than one thing at the same time mentally, as a mental juggler. You are simultaneously able to keep a task or question in mind while working on the solution or answers. You listen to yourself as you proceed, integrating what you feel inside your mind with what you experience outside yourself, moving back and forth between the inner and outer experiences.
- You sense rhythm well and are readily able to move from one thought to another without losing track of the various strands of the rhythm. You continuously sense them. This has a lot to do with being an analog processor of information who has strong rhythmic intelligence.
- You become so absorbed in what you're doing that you take on its language and follow the direction it takes you rather than superimposing your own structure on the task, thus limiting its potential growth. You *become one* with the task—a very Zen way of being.
- Because of your style of brain construction, you can count on it to produce solutions to problems by simply introducing the problem and then letting go to allow a solution to present itself. You don't have to purposely "think it through." In fact, such purposeful thought can block successful outcomes from your style of problem-solving. You simply need to let your way do its job out of your conscious awareness.

Problems You Face Because You Create in Your Mind:

- You may discount your thinking because it falls outside the standard way of working through a problem or creating something new.
- Your way of thinking and doing may be judged as less valuable than the standard linear way of achieving information.

Your Goal:

Learn to use the style of working and creating that is the way of the True You.

What Not To Do:

Do not discount your inner process or judge it to have less value than more mechanistic or linear processes. Do not try to work from a tight plan that leaves no room for creative thought to emerge.

Your Work:

1. Know that your way of handling information and finding answers is a tangible process with which you are blessed by virtue of your brain construction. Yours is a variation within the realm of human physiological potential.
   I may need to change the way I've thought about my thinking. _____yes.
   The change will look like this: _____
   _____ .

2. Rejoice in your wonderful skills.
   I can now be happy with my way of handling information and finding answers. _____yes

3. To learn to use your special thinking skills, practice being aware of what you're feeling as you proceed in a task. Pay attention to the situations where your creative thinking skills emerge. Compare these situations and note how and when they are strongest.
   I am thinking of a time recently when I was faced with a need to find solutions to a project. When I think back I realize that I was feeling _____
   _____ .

I can also think of other situations when my creative thinking skills emerged. _____yes

When I compare these situations and note how and when they were strongest, I find_____

_____.

4. Note analogies that pop into your mind and your level of comfort with the environment in which you find/found yourself. The analogies that popped in my mind in the same situation were _____

_____.

I also realize I felt _____with the environment in which I found myself.

5. Notice your comfort with the types of people you're around when you become most creative.

When I think of the types of people I am around when I feel the most creative, they can best be described as _____

_____.

6. Note what you can do to replicate or create states of mind in the future that please you. Work that is open ended and free of rigid requirements is likely to elicit your creativity.

In the future I realize I can _____

_____ to create a state of mind to be creative.

7. Environments that you like will more readily spawn creative achievement on your part. You are likely to find that warm, receptive, open-minded, creative people encourage your flowering productions.

I become most creative in environments that are _____

_____.

And the people I most like to be around in order to be creative are _____

_____.

8. Keep as much track of your experiences as any researcher does. This does not mean that you have to create a linear database on paper, but it means that you create a mental recall system. When something you do doesn't fit into the schema that has begun to emerge in relation to your creative activity, question it, find out what is different from when something does fit. You'll figure out the differences, and they will end up making good sense to you. And you'll have learned more about yourself.

When I think of a creative situation with
which I've worked, I am beginning to
see what fit and what didn't.   _____yes

The next time I am in a creative mode, I will
watch carefully for the patterns and
schema that are emerging.   _____yes

I'll question what I sense or see, and I'll find
out what is different about it from when it fits. _____yes

9. Give yourself permission to move in directions your senses draw you toward, rather than trying to purposely figure out what the next step *should* be.

I now give myself permission to move in directions my senses draw me toward. _____yes

10. Be careful of losing belief in your process. Suppose one day you aren't feeling well. Or maybe someone purposely or inadvertently pressures you into working in a more linear fashion than is right for you, and you get off track. Your creativity bites the dust and you wonder if you can count on it. That undermines your confidence in yourself and pulls your focus from your inner process to an external one.

Reassure yourself that your way does work. Get quiet. Ask your inner self to again show you the way, and you will find that your unique guidance system reasserts itself. You'll again see your mental pictures and have your spontaneous insights and solutions.

I hereby commit, if I've been drawn off track from my way of doing things, to get quiet and ask my inner self to again show me the way. I know I will be shown it and will reconnect with my unique guidance system. _____yes

11. Be cautious about whom you talk with in relation to the way you work. Many people may not have the brain construction to work in the way that you do or even understand it. Unfortunately, they may believe that their way is the superior or right way. Their approach can make you feel unnecessarily unsure of yourself.

I absolutely will use caution with regard to whom I share my style of thinking with. _____yes

12. Do not hesitate to back off from a path that is not producing or for which you have no enthusiasm.

I commit to back off from a path that is not
producing for me.   _____yes

I commit to back off from a path for which I have
   no enthusiasm. _____yes

13. Try a new direction or new angle whenever you want,
   whether it makes logical sense or not. It *will* end up working for you.
   I commit to try a new direction or new angle whenever I want.
   _____yes

14. If your creative mind works too fast for comfort, check your
   environment to be sure you're not feeding your mind too
   much stimulation. This can happen when you get talking to
   another creative person or are working on a team.
   I will remember to check my environment and the people in
   it when my mind gets working too fast to be effective.
   _____yes

15. Reduce the stimulation that surrounds you. This may mean
   you need to go off by yourself to work for a while.
   I will reduce the stimulation around me and may go off for
   a while to work in solitude. _____yes

16. Consider putting yourself on a schedule and cut out extra-
   neous activities when you are on a creative roll. This may
   mean letting the dishes go or the lawn grow an inch higher.
   It sure means you need to avoid problem-solving and brainstorming meetings or discussions.
   If I'm overstimulated, I'll cut out activities
      that are overstimulating.   _____yes
   I will also avoid problem-solving and
      brainstorming meetings for the time being.   _____yes

17. You may also find your mind works overtime for emotional
   reasons, if you have a hidden emotional agenda. Doubt
   about what you are doing or guilt that you're doing some-
   thing wrong will cause undue stress.
   If my mind is working overtime for emotional
      reasons, I will analyze my feelings.
   Am I feeling doubt?   _____yes
   Am I feeling guilt?   _____yes
   Am I feeling any other feelings?   _____yes

18. Deal with your emotional stress before proceeding with your
   project agenda. If you're feeling doubt, ask yourself some
   questions.
   Where is the feeling coming from? _____
   _____
   From whom did I learn the feeling? _____

19. Once you've established the source of the feeling, take your courage in hand and take a stand, returning the doubt to its original source. Then follow your commitment.

    If guilt has intruded, also recall from whom you learned it. Take your power back as you revisit the value system you wish to live by at this time. (See "Deciding What to Do" in the epilogue.)

    I take my courage in hand and will take a stand, returning doubt to its original source. _____yes

    I learned guilt from _____.

    I take my power back.   _____yes

    I revisit the value system I wish to live by at
       this time.   _____yes

20. If you have multiple creative and imaginative scenarios spinning in your head, make a list of the various projects and scenarios. Then make a folder for each.

    I have _____ scenarios spinning in my head. Here is a list of the various projects and scenarios:

    _____   _____

    _____   _____

    _____   _____

    _____   _____

21. Pick one to focus on now. It doesn't matter which one you choose. Let your heart be your guide.

    I will focus on _____.

22. Promise yourself you'll work with each project in turn, *one at a time*.

    I promise to work on each project in turn, leaving none out as long as my heart is touched by the project or idea. _____yes

23. Go to work, paying attention to the project you've chosen.

    I will go to work and concentrate my attention on the one project I've chosen. _____yes

24. When other ideas intrude into your thinking, write them down and put them into the folder where they belong or make a new folder for new ideas. Do not pursue the ideas further *at this time*.

    I will place any intruding thought onto paper and put it into a folder for later attention. _____yes

25. Realize that you'll never run out of ideas. And know you'll never totally lose an idea. Even if you don't use it in its present form, it will recycle to reappear as a part of another idea. You will not suffer a loss.

I know I'll never run out of ideas nor will I lose any. My ideas are safe. _____yes

26. Enjoy the wonderful mind that is a part of the True You.
I happily enjoy my wonderful mind. _____yes

Your Commitments:

I commit to honor the way in which I am naturally
constructed.   _____yes
I commit to be good to myself and learn all I can
about using the brain that is mine to its optimal level. _____yes

What Makes This Hard To Do:

Western culture tends to judge thinking styles, placing them into preferred categories as if there were a single way to look at things. Moving into the "flow" or process of how something works means you may have to go against the grain.

Generally, fear that you won't pick the right project also makes it hard to trust your creative thinking process. Such fear may slow you from making the choice of which project/idea/direction to pursue. In reality, it doesn't matter which one you choose. Basically you'll end up being you, expressing your creative self and creating something that will be wonderful that will please you.

You will have to learn to believe in yourself and surround yourself with supportive people.

SUCCEEDING AS A CREATIVE EMPLOYEE

Question:

Do you have trouble working for people who require you to do things their way?

Why This Happens:

- Your mental style does not fit your supervisor's management style. As a creative person you are guided from within, marching, as they say, to your own drum. You are a responsible person who is more than willing to take control of any work project in which you believe, but can't tolerate direction from someone who doesn't think as you do.

- Because you have an inner guiding light that is sensitively attuned to your creative mood, one that is intricately interwoven to your heart's desires, you always know what fits you. And that makes you feel good. You also know what is not part of your innate life's agenda. Trying to work on something that doesn't fit you makes you feel awful, enough so that you may feel you can't stand it another minute.

- You have a wonderful sense of natural timing that works for you. It is uneven, causing you to work a lot one day and not much another, but you have a clear sense of project time lines. You simply don't break time up in a systematic way. That's not the way your analog-processing mind orders time. You order time by the content of what you're doing and the feelings within yourself.

- Given a problem to solve, your creative mind will immediately go to work finding a solution. You will move to your own rhythm. Probably you'll be keeping the end goal in sight throughout.

- But when someone requires you to use their steps, their rhythm, and their timing, you are likely to not only dislike the task but also fail to do the task well. As a responsible person you will sense the lack of fit and probably become angry and experience a high level of stress. As a result you may begin to lose your commitment to your job. In turn, you will no longer be able to act responsibly, which in and of itself will cause you more stress. A vicious cycle will have been set in motion. Depression is not unlikely and your self-esteem will suffer.

Problems You Face Succeeding as a Creative Employee:

- Your work productivity is interrupted and your goals are thwarted when your supervisor or your job requirements don't fit.
- You may start avoiding work, hating your job, and get into trouble with your boss if he/she is expecting things from you that don't fit your brainstyle.
- You may face the need for major change in your life.

Your Goal:

To put yourself in a work situation that fits you and allows you to use your creativity.

What Not To Do:

Neither compromise your mental health nor allow yourself to act in a way that makes you less than proud and happy with yourself.

Your Work:

1. Assess your situation. Think about the last time you were happy on the job. Check the fit of your brain construction and your personality with the duties, pacing, and creative freedom attached to the job at that time.
   My brain construction is _____ .
   My personality is _____ .
   The requirements of my job with regard to duties, pacing, and creative freedom when I was happy were _____
   _____ .
   The requirements of my job with regard to duties, pacing, and creative freedom now require _____
   _____
   _____ .

2. Note what's changed. Be as specific and detailed as you can. You may find that telling someone the details that surrounded any change will help you recall small bits of information that will hold the key to your understanding your situation.
   I will ask _____ to listen to my comparison.

3. Ask the person listening to be on the lookout for shifts in your expression. Your feelings will reflect what started going wrong and be expressed on your face and through your body language.
I will ask _____ to watch for shifts in my facial expression and body language as I speak of different job requirements and how well they fit me. He/She reports the following: _____

_____

_____ .

4. Spend some time comparing what you want to do in relation to responsibilities you choose to honor. Ask yourself:
Am I responsible for meeting my basic
   survival needs and those of my family?   _____yes _____no
At this time, am I able to take the time
   sto eek work in which I can express
   my creativity?   _____yes _____no
Once my basic needs are met, how do I feel about spending time expressing my creativity? _____

_____ .

At this time in my life, do I value my need for status
   and appearances more than my need to express
   my creativity?   _____yes _____no
Do my values reflect my talents
   and desires?   _____yes _____no
Is my decision heartfelt or logical? _____

5. Look practically at the commitments and obligations you have at this time. This will include family, debt, and other involvements. Check to see the length of time you can anticipate the obligations to last. Be cautious that you don't automatically accept past decisions and current involvements as obligations that are unchangeable.

   For example, suppose you have lived in the same neighborhood for many years and assumed that your kids would graduate from high school there. But now that you're miserable on your job, you need to be sure that you still feel the same way about where to live, because you might need to move.

   If you have a child who is a high school senior, you may decide this is definitely not a time to move. But if your kids are younger or older and perhaps are at a transition time in their lives, you and your family may realize you can make a change that will be a whole lot better for you and one that will not hurt them.

Currently, I have the following obligations: _____
_____ .
But I see that I may want to rethink the following ones:
_____
_____ .

6. Hold a family meeting and share what is happening to you at work. Share your feelings. Ask for observations and input from everyone, your spouse and kids alike.

When my family held a family meeting, we found out _____
_____
_____ .

7. Then decide with your spouse whether a change to something that fits you better is in order as soon as possible or whether you will make the best of the situation for the time being, promising yourself a change later. If you choose the latter, find ways to use your creativity on the job or outside of work—ways that bring you in touch with your heart and bring hope into your life.

It appears that a change is a good idea at this time. _____yes
It appears that it would be better to wait to make a change. _____yes
I can think of several ways to use my creativity if I stay on the job for the time being. _____
_____ .

8. If you stay with the job, look for opportunities to transfer to a different boss or ask for autonomy with regard to parts of your work.

I might be able to do _____
_____ .

9. Keep reminding yourself that your situation is temporary and that you will stand by your creative nature. Stay alert to opportunities that will bring you a better fit.

Indeed, I am aware that my situation is
temporary.   _____yes
I look out for opportunities that better fit me
and my personal needs and choices.   _____yes

Your Commitments:

I am committed to my family.	_____yes
I am committed to my creative self.	_____yes
I am committed to finding the right environment to support my creativity fully.	_____yes

What Makes This Hard To Do:

The hardest part of succeeding as a creative employee is failing to believe in yourself and losing hope that you'll ever feel happy and genuinely productive again. That's your battle. Rise to the occasion, and you will be happy and productive once more.

Epilogue

Throughout my writing, I've shared much of what I've personally learned and professionally observed over many years. The more I've learned, the more I've come to realize the importance of honoring human diversity, for that builds the broadest foundation for healthy living in a wholesome society. As each of us plays the role we are best suited to play, we add a unique ingredient to the mix of any achievement, dream, or goal we value.

The wiser I've become, the more I have come to value the intrinsic potential each of us has within ourselves to know what is right for ourselves. Truly, no one else knows as well as you do what fits you, so you can use your natural talents and skills to their maximum. Yet I've repeatedly seen disconnection from that inner knowing as a person is taught what he or she *needs* to do, how he or she *should* be, or what he or she *ought* to want.

Often shared in well-meaning ways, these *shoulds* and *oughts* break the connection you have with your True Self—the vehicle that knows how to bring your potential to its peak level of performance.

Finally, the more self-aware I've become and the stronger I've grown emotionally, the more I realize the effect each of us can have on the direction our lives take. As you believe, so you create. These are not empty words. The power of belief to affect outcomes is only beginning to be understood and acknowledged. We are a long way from harnessing that power. And we each have much emotional work to do to get beyond the self-imposed limitations created by our fears, doubts, and disbelief in this power that is available to each of us. But we are learning to use the power of belief for the valuable expression of our True Selves.

To achieve the success that benefits both ourselves and the society in which we live, we must fully honor our True Selves, scrupulously engaging, whenever possible, in what fits our makeup: our style of brain construction, our personalities, and our interests and heartfelt desires.

We must gently and knowingly encourage the parts of our behavior and emotions that have been hurt, healing our Wounded Selves.

And, when necessary, we must make sure we do not further wound ourselves as our Accommodating Selves strive to live and learn in today's world.

I'd like to end this book with two additional suggestions for applying the ADD way of thinking. One is entitled "Deciding What to Do." It highlights the reasons why it's hard to honor what we want, caught instead in the trap of trying to do what we think we *should* do. And it gives you steps to consider that will allow you to marry your thinking with your desire and to respect and express your True Self by doing what you want to do, not what you *should* do.

The second and final application will guide you in relation to enhancing your ability to use the power inherent in what you believe. Then, as you choose, you can purposely create a life of your own making by becoming aware of what you believe and using that belief to create the outcomes you desire.

In *The New ADD in Adults Workbook*, I leave you with that which I've garnered from my journey. I intend for it to be helpful and empowering to you. I also encourage you to take only what fits you. Honor your own timing and only select the parts to which you are drawn. Above all, know that I respect and value the True You. With confidence I release my words into your care.

DECIDING WHAT TO DO

Question:

Do you have trouble deciding to let yourself do what you'd really like to do?

Why This Happens:

- You are being swayed by what you *should* do rather than following the lead of what you *want* to do. This means your behavior is driven by *shoulds*. A *should* is a belief—that is, something you were *taught* at an earlier time by someone else. A belief's power lies in the fact that you learned it when you were very young and were dependent on those around you who were guiding your behavior. Because of this powerful early learning—learning that is often forgotten by all of us when we grow older—we tend to think what we believe is *the only way* to think. That is why beliefs are hard to change.
- The words *should* and *ought* continue to carry a strong legacy from early years, so much so that you tend to revert to feeling dependent when they are used.
- When you do something you don't think you *should* do, you will tend to feel *guilty*. When you do something you don't *want* to do, you'll feel *resentful*. Either way, you feel bad.
- As a result, the *shoulds* control your life. But they also cheat you of your life. They may pull you away from acting in behalf of your True Self. They may separate you from what you love. They control your actions, driving you to act in ways that may not be good for you.
- When what you have been taught doesn't fit you naturally, you will become conflicted and unable to know what to do. You will have a hard time making decisions. This is because there is a strong drive within all of us to live in alignment with our True Selves. This drive feels like *desire* and *wanting* while a belief in *shoulds* confuses you, creating feelings of hesitation, guilt, and resentment.

Problems You Face Deciding What To Do:

- Dealing with reality.
- Others putting down your dreams and desires.

- Being judged and criticized for wanting to follow your desires and dreams.
- Feeling guilty, trapped, depressed, and paralyzed.

Your Goal:

To align your belief systems and behavior with the True You.

What Not To Do:

Do not fail to align your belief systems with the True You.

Your Work:

1. Rethink the beliefs you were taught at an earlier time so you can decide if you want to keep them or not.
   I commit to bring what I believe into conscious awareness and rethink these beliefs in order to decide if I want to keep them or not. _____yes
2. Ask yourself what the belief is that is causing you conflict—that is, "What do I think I *should* do?" Consider, for example, the belief, "I *should* stay home with my child and do my housework."
   When I consider following my dreams and desires, I believe

   _____

   _____ .
3. Ask yourself, "From whom did I learn this belief?" Watch for snippets of thoughts, memories, mental pictures, and conversations in your mind. They are likely to reflect the settings in which you learned the belief. You may instantly recall the exact person from whom you learned it. Or your learning may have occurred in a more subtle way as you sensed what many people around you believed, even if they never said anything directly to you.
   I learned my belief from _____ .
4. Next, ask yourself if you practiced the belief so you would be praised and feel accepted. Or did you adhere to the guidelines of the belief because you were afraid not to do so? Disapproval may have created feelings of fear if you are a sensitive person. Of course, you might also have been afraid of being punished if you didn't follow the dictates of the belief.

I was praised and accepted when I followed the
   belief(s) I was taught.   _____yes
I adhered to guidelines of the belief because I
   was afraid not to do so.   _____yes

5. If you suffer from the fear of repercussions when you don't do
   what someone else wants, begin to build your independence
   and courage to stand up for what *you* think is right. Use the
   pronoun "I" liberally. You might say, "*I* make decisions based
   on what *I* know about myself. *I* am in charge of myself."
   I am willing to gather my courage to stand up for what *I*
   think is right. _____yes _____I am not ready to do this.

6. Next, check to see what new information you have obtained
   that you didn't have previously. For example, you now know
   that brain diversity affects what each individual does. You
   may realize that there is no *one right way* for everyone.
   As I've grown older I realize that there is no
      one right way for everyone.   _____yes
   I didn't know this when I was young, so now
      I feel differently about what I believe is right
      in many areas.   _____yes

7. Notice the effects of trying to do something that doesn't fit
   you but that you feel you *should* do. Perhaps feelings of resentment come to mind, or guilty feelings or depression or
   anger. Simply note them. You will come to realize that you
   don't have to continue to feel any of these when you rework
   your belief system to fit the True You while you continue to
   live a caring, responsible life.
   The effects I feel when I try to fit into ways of doing things
   that compromise my True Self are _____
   _____.

8. Now decide what you want to believe. You may either adopt
   a new belief or continue your previous one. If you continue
   the previous one, it now is one that belongs to you because
   you've thought through it. It's no longer a *should*. You've
   made it your own by choosing it with your adult mind and
   heart working in unison.
   I choose to keep the previous belief I had, but now it is mine.
      _____yes
   Apply this to any belief you choose to consider.

9. You may decide you want to modify your previous belief
   based on the new information you've obtained. For example,

using the example of a young mother, you might decide you are going to give yourself permission to get a job doing what you love because the other course simply doesn't work for you. You become creative about how to use your time with your child. You make sure you have a job with flexibility so you can be available to your child at special times.

You decide to spend some of your wages on housecleaning services. You might even decide to take a few extra hours so you can pay for yard work, too.

Again referring to the young mother, the nice part about her work with her values is that she gets what fits her while still being a responsible person. And her child gets a fulfilled parent who can teach her child how to also live up to his or her natural self.

I choose to change the previous belief that I held. _____yes

I know that it is okay to consider any beliefs I have in this way, choosing or rejecting that belief. I am pleased that I have the ability to think for myself. _____yes

Your Commitments:

I commit to rethink my values one at a time.   _____yes
When I feel it is right and valuable to change one,
   I will do that.   _____yes
When I choose to retain an initial value, I commit
   to do that.   _____yes

What Makes This Hard To Do:

Because beliefs are initially learned when we are very young and de-pendent and have black-and-white thinking, we tend to feel they are cast in concrete. We may not question them, much less think to change them, even though our thinking has matured to take on the gray cast of adult life.

BUILDING A LIFE ACCORDING TO WHAT YOU BELIEVE

Question:

Do you struggle to believe positively about your True Self?

Why This Happens:

- You may have learned you're okay no matter what your race, religion, sex, sexual preference, age, or interests. These all fall under the rubric of diversity. But diversity in brainstyles has not yet achieved equivalent status.
- In a society that has historically struggled with diversity, anyone who is not like the model held up as the preferred way to be is considered inadequate until that group of people refuses to be seen as lesser any longer.
- Any preferred model is a mental construct, an illusion that sees one kind of person as perfect.
- But every attribute of brainstyle has strengths and weaknesses. Each strength has a down side and each weakness has an up side.
- Some of your characteristics that have been shaped by your style of brain construction will be favored by the cultural model under which you live. Others won't no matter what your unique style.
- In reality, there is absolutely nothing *wrong* with you no matter what your style of brain construction. To the degree to which you have been constantly placed in environments that don't fit you, taught in ways that don't fit your brainstyle, and had expectations made of you that fail to take brainstyle diversity into account, you have been wounded. You may *feel* there is something wrong with you when, in reality, you've simply been hurt by living in a mis-fitting environment. The True You is just fine.
- This myth was passed on to our generation and is being perpetuated to future generations. What we believe we create. We now have a chance to stop wasting human potential for ourselves and our children and our children's children as diversity of brainstyle is recognized for what it is.

Problems You Face Building a Life According to What You Believe:

- You fear your ability to build a better life because of past failures.
- You fear there is something wrong with you and fear that there isn't something wrong with you that could be fixed.
- You feel sad and confused.

Your Goal:

To accept the power you have to create a self-image that is positive and yields constructive results for you and the world around you while honoring the unique attributes that make you up.

What Not To Do:

Do not believe you are anything less that wonderful *as you are.*

Your Work:

1. Remember the way in which you view yourself affects not only how you feel about yourself, but how and what you are able to do in your life. It affects your behavior.
   I know that the way I view myself affects how
     I feel about myself.   _____yes
   I know that how and what I am able to do
     in my life is affected by how I view myself.   _____yes
   And these affect my behavior.   _____yes
2. Remember, you have the power to create a positive self-image by accepting the unique combination of brainstyle attributes you possess. You can affirm this by saying, "I create a positive self-image of myself. I see myself as fine, just the way I am made."
   I will write and then repeat the above statement. _____
   _____
   _____
3. Become self-aware of your brainstyle without judging it.
   I know my brainstyle is _____ .
4. Become aware of the learning and working and living environments that suit the way in which your brain is constructed.

I commit to become aware of the learning and working and living environments that suit the way in which my brain is constructed. _____yes

5. Affirm your desire to fit into those environments. You can say, "I desire to find the environments in which to learn, work, and live—environments that naturally fit me."
I will write and then repeat the above statement. _____

_____

_____

_____ .

6. Support and nurture parts of yourself that have been hurt because of a lack of understanding of brain diversity. Identify behavior that is the result of a poor self-belief and target it for change. Counseling, hypnotherapy, and/or prayer may be useful in doing this.
I commit to support and nurture the parts of myself that have been hurt because of a lack of understanding of brain diversity. _____yes
I have the following behavior that results in poor self-belief:

_____

_____

_____ .

I commit to target this behavior for change. _____yes
I plan to use the following means to change my behavior:

_____

_____

_____ .

7. When you are ready, forgive those who judged and hurt you because of the way your brain is constructed, for they knew and know not what they do. You do not need to rush this step. Take your time.
I _____am _____am not ready to forgive those who hurt me.
If I am not ready now, I will reconsider at a later time. _____yes

8. Build bridges to environments that don't fit you without judging yourself or the environments. Say, "I build a bridge to any environment in which I find myself, even though I and my environment utilize different brainstyles."
I will carefully build bridges to environments
    that don't fit me.   _____yes

I will not judge myself or the environment.   _____yes

I will say, _____

_____ .

9. Consider mentoring others so they can see themselves as valuable, while teaching them to effectively use the skills their brainstyle provides them.

    I am interested in mentoring others. _____yes

10. Refuse to accept current terms that *pathologize* your *condition*.

    I refuse to accept terms that *pathologize* and *medicalize* my style of brain construction. _____yes

11. Consider becoming active in changing the perception of people who have brainstyle attributes that do not fit the standardized social model. This means working to see that every child receives an education that fits him or her. Equal educational opportunity for all people regardless of brain diversity is critical. Equal opportunity means that a person's ability to do a job or show what he or she knows is assessed in ways that reflect his or her style of brain construction. It means standing up against professionals who say differently.

    As the perception of the public is heightened, the major diversity issue of the twenty-first century will be successfully put to rest as all styles of brain construction are equally honored and allowed to function.

    I am interested in becoming active in changing the perception of people who have brainstyle attributes that do not fit the standardized social model. _____yes

12. Learn the language of those with a different style of brain construction from yours.

    I will look for opportunities to spend time with people with a different style of brain construction than I have in an attempt to reach better understanding. _____yes

13. Learn how to team up with those who are different so that goals can be reached and growth achieved in balanced ways.

    I will look for opportunities to team up with someone with a brainstyle different from mine. _____yes

Your Commitments:

I commit to become all I can become, honoring
my True Self.   _____yes
I commit to protecting and healing my Wounded Self.   _____yes
I commit to supporting and guiding my
Accommodating Self so that I can avoid further
wounding on my way to becoming all I am
capable of becoming.   _____yes
I commit to work with others, honoring different
brainstyles in the best interest of all of us.   _____yes

What Makes This Hard To Do:

Changing beliefs is one of the hardest jobs anyone can tackle.

Addendum: The Americans with Disabilities Act

- You must realize that what you need to get through school is an equal opportunity to learn what you're capable of learning and to prove you know it.
- Currently, that means you will need to turn to the Americans with Disabilities Act. This act says that if you have the intelligence to learn a subject but have some learning difficulties that get in the way of applying that intelligence, you must be given reasonable accommodation so you can succeed.
- You need to go to the Special Services Office at the college in which you are enrolled or intend to enroll to initiate the process and determine your eligibility. You can do this even before classes start.
- To formally acquire ADA accommodation, you must undergo an assessment of your intellectual capability. You must also be assessed with regard to your "handicapping condition." If there is sufficient discrepancy between these two assessments, you are "diagnosed" with what is called a learning disability. Many of the difficulties kinesthetic, big-picture people have in school lead to the assignment of a learning disabilities label such as ADD or ADHD. With this label, you can apply for special services at your school of choice.

The testing must be done by a licensed professional such as a psychologist or psychiatrist. Sometimes an educational diagnostician's or counselor's testing is acceptable.

- Many college offices are now working with professors and students in an attempt to provide learner-friendly approaches and materials for all students without the need of formal testing.
- Some of the services available include:
  - Unlimited test-taking time
  - A quiet area, free of distraction, in which to take tests
  - Tests designed to support the brainstyle construction of students—that is, essays, projects, or oral exams, instead of multiple-choice or fill-in-the-blank formats
  - Assignment of a note taker
  - Assistance in outlining main points in class and textbook material
  - Use of a tape recorder during lectures
  - One-on-one tutoring
  - Front-row seating
  - Priority use of computer resources designed to help students with organization and study skills
  - Access to recorded versions of textbooks
  - Assistance in creating a structured time schedule
  - Assistance in developing priorities for long-term projects
  - Assistance in relating to authority figures
  - Assistance in translating differences in brainstyles
  - Substitution of a required class by one that isn't compromised because of the learning differences

These are only some of the services available. A student may request any reasonable accommodation.

- You need to know that you can request these accommodations whether you're formally identified as learning disabled or as someone with an ADD style of brain construction not favored in school. More and more college teachers, especially at the community college level, are responding to student's learning needs.
- However, without a formal diagnosis, the faculty is not *mandated* to provide what you need.

What Makes This Hard To Do:

You must be honest with yourself and not attempt to use ADA so that you can study subject matter that is not suited to your overall capability.

ADA requires you to say that you are "disabled," but in reality that is a misnomer. What you need is simply the opportunity to do your work in a way that fits you. Ultimately, this right will be seen as the diversity issue that it is and, as a result, will fall under equal opportunities legislation. Then you will not have to say you're handicapped in order to be given the opportunity to get an education or do your job. But for now, ADA can make a difference in your life.

Other Titles Published by Lynn Weiss, Ph.D.

Attention Deficit Disorder in Adults, 4th ed.
View from the Cliff: A Course in Achieving Daily Focus
A.D.D. and Success
A.D.D. and Creativity
Give Your A.D.D. Teen a Chance
A.D.D. on the Job
The Attention Deficit Disorder in Adults Workbook
Attention Deficit Disorder in Adults:
Practical Help and Understanding

About the Author

A psychotherapist for forty years, **Lynn Weiss** has an extensive backgroud in training, teaching, program development, and writing about human behavior and child development. For the past two decades, she's concentrated on forwarding an enlightened perspective on Attention Deficit Disorder as a brainstyle diversity issue.

Clinically trained through a NIMH clinical fellowship at the University of Washington Medical School, Dr. Weiss has brought her education to a practical level that builds from the health and strength in those with whom she comes in contact. She currently is writing non-fiction and fiction for adults and children and doing program development for natural resource managers as well as A.D.D. from her home in the woods in Central Texas.